Dyslexia: A Parents' and Teachers' Guide

PARENTS' and TEACHERS' GUIDES

Series Editor
Professor Colin Baker, *University of Wales, Bangor, Wales, Great Britain*

Second Language Students in Mainstream Classrooms
  COREEN SEARS

Other Books of Interest
Building Bridges: Multilingual Resources for Children
  MULTILINGUAL RESOURCES FOR CHILDREN PROJECT
Children Talking: The Development of Pragmatic Competence
  LINDA THOMPSON (ed.)
Computers and Talk in the Primary Classroom
  RUPERT WEGERIF and PETER SCRIMSHAW (eds.)
The Guided Construction of Knowledge
  NEIL MERCER
Encyclopedia of Bilingual Education and Bilingualism
  COLIN BAKER and SYLVIA PRYS JONES
Learning about Punctuation
  NIGEL HALL and ANNE ROBINSON (eds)
A Parents' and Teachers' Guide to Bilingualism
  COLIN BAKER
Worlds of Literacy
  M. HAMILTON, D. BARTON and R. IVANIC (eds)

Please contact us for the latest book information:
Multilingual Matters, Frankfurt Lodge, Clevedon Hall
Victoria Road, Clevedon, BS21 7HH, England
http:/www.multilingual-matters.com

PARENTS' AND TEACHER' GUIDES 3
Series Editor: Colin Baker

Dyslexia
A Parents' and Teachers' Guide

Trevor Payne and Elizabeth Turner

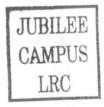

MULTILINGUAL MATTERS LTD
Clevedon • Philadelphia • Toronto • Sydney • Johannesburg

Library of Congress Cataloging in Publication Data

Payne, Trevor
Dyslexia: A Parents' and Teachers' Guide/Trevor Payne and Elizabeth Turner
Parents' and Teachers' Guides: 3
Includes bibliographical references and index
1. Dyslexic children–Education. 2. Learning. 3. Dyslexic children–Legal status, laws, etc.–Great
Britain. I. Turner, Elizabeth. II. Title. III. Series: Parents' and teachers' guides: no. 3.
LC4710.G7P39   1998
371.91'44–dc21   98-27057

British Library Cataloguing in Publication Data

A CIP catalogue record for this book is available from the British Library.

ISBN 1-85359-411-3 (hbk)
ISBN 1-85359-410-5 (pbk)

1004781010

Multilingual Matters Ltd

UK: Frankfurt Lodge, Clevedon Hall, Victoria Road, Clevedon BS21 7HH.
USA: 325 Chestnut Street, Philadelphia, PA 19106, USA.
Canada: 5201 Dufferin Street, North York, Ontario M3H 5T8, Canada.
Australia: P.O. Box 586, Artamon, NSW, Australia.
South Africa: PO Box 1080, Northcliffe 2115, Johannesburg, South Africa.

Typeset by Bookcraft, Stroud.
Printed and bound in Great Britain by WBC Book Manufacturers Ltd.

Contents

Acknowledgements

We are indebted to Professor Colin Baker of the University of Bangor for his unstinting advice, support and encouragement during the writing of this book. We would also like to thank, for their help and support, the following:

Chris Harvey, Headteacher of Hawarden High School

Keith McDonogh, Director of Education, Libraries and Information for Flintshire

Michael Payne, for drawing the cartoons

All the dyslexic children we have taught over the years.

Dedication

This book is dedicated to:

Sarah and Nicholas whose dyslexic struggles and successes are my inspiration and motivation, and to Stewart for constant support and encouragement.   ET

My wife, Lynwen and my children, Christopher, Matthew and Michael, for sharing me with a word-processor over the last two years and to my father, David, who left school at fourteen but has never stopped learning — and lecturing — since.   TP

Chapter 1
Introduction

This chapter contains a brief overview of children with specific learning difficulties (dyslexia). The book is first placed in context with others written on the
same subject. Then the main themes and contents are introduced. A working
definition of dyslexia is given along with an indication of its main effects on
children's ability to thrive in school. We do not dwell on the theory of dyslexia. That task is for others. The chapter finishes with a brief guide to the
book itself.

What Do We Call It?

The learning difficulty commonly known as 'dyslexia' has different names
depending on who you speak to and where. In Britain, the officially recognised term
for dyslexia is now settled as being 'specific learning difficulties (dyslexia)'. This
expression is rather cumbersome for us to repeat it in full as often as it occurs in this
book. Therefore, for our and our reader's ease, we have shortened it to 'dyslexia'
and to children experiencing the condition as 'dyslexic children' or 'children with
dyslexia'. Thus, when we say children are 'dyslexic' we mean they are experiencing
'specific learning difficulties (dyslexia)'. When we refer to 'dyslexia', we mean that
we are saying something about 'specific learning difficulties (dyslexia)'.

Main Aim of This Book

An acceptance of dyslexia has now acquired recognition in our schools, colleges
and universities. Our knowledge of its causes, effects and remediation are continually developing. There is a huge and ever-growing body of information and opinion
on the subject. This book does not attempt to be an encyclopaedic account of this
knowledge. We wrote the book with the following readers in mind:

- parents of dyslexic children or adults who may be dyslexic;

- teachers in training;

- newly qualified teachers;

- class or subject teachers who have little or no specialist knowledge in the field.

Our aim is to give our readers the information they need to better help the dyslexic child or children in front of them. These children will benefit best from

informed support. In doing so we have assumed little previous knowledge of the subject. We have concentrated only on providing you with the information which you need to know. We have tried to convey this information in language which is as jargon free as we could possibly make it. We have not attempted to break new ground or provide a new rationale for dyslexia, in a way which would be of interest to specialist teachers or psychologists or other 'experts'.

References

To make the book more readable we have not used academic references of the type:

Brown (1988) stated that . . .

or

The main arguments for this theory were put forward by Smith *et al* (1997).

However, we have used many sources of written information. Where we are dealing with knowledge which we believe is broadly accepted by almost everyone in the field and which has been written up by many authors, we have not made specific reference to them in the text. These sources are accredited in the booklist. However, where we refer to an idea or a technique which is very distinctly the work of one person or group of people, we have named that person.

Conflicting Views

As far as possible we have tried to restrict ourselves to those features of dyslexia about which there is a consensus. However, there is still some disagreement among experts about many aspects of the subject. This is true even at the level of its exact causes and the best ways it may be overcome. While this may seem inevitable for what is still a relatively new field of study, it can be very confusing for the 'non-expert'. Therefore, we have mainly restricted ourselves to knowledge about which there is a general agreement. An example of this is the desirability for dyslexic children to be taught using multi-sensory techniques (i.e. learning through more than one sense). Nearly everyone in the field seems to agree that these techniques are effective for most dyslexic children.

We could not avoid controversy completely. There are some areas of difference which we had to address and clearly state our own position. Such areas are important to parents and teachers. For instance, you may be aware of the debate about teaching methods which centres around the use of 'real books' as against 'phonics' to assist children to become readers. As we were writing the book, this debate was being refuelled by an apparent assumption on the part of the incoming Labour Government that a heavy emphasis on phonic instruction is essential for reading tuition. This view is shared by many in the dyslexia field, who are passionate in their belief that the use of real-book methods has hindered the reading development of many children. We do not wholly subscribe to this view. We believe that poor teaching of reading using the real-book methods may have this effect but that poor phonics teaching is equally unproductive. Our view is that real-book methods, used properly in combination with other methods, including phonics, are very appropriate means for dyslexic children to learn to read. This is dealt with fully in Chapter 2.

What are Specific Learning Difficulties (Dyslexia)?

Nearly every book on dyslexia starts by saying that dyslexia is defined in many different ways. This profusion of definitions needs explaining. The main cause probably lies in the number of different professionals who become involved in working with dyslexic children. These include doctors, psychologists, linguists and teachers. Each profession will approach the subject from a different perspective. General Practitioners mainly deal with physical ailments. It is not surprising then that if you ask a doctor to define dyslexia you will probably get an answer which describes it in terms of the brain's physical structure. In contrast, many Educational Psychologists, trained in the ways children use and acquire information, will approach dyslexia by concentrating on how dyslexic children learn. Similarly a linguist will probably define dyslexia in terms of children's language skills. Teachers though, who actually have to do something about it in the classroom, will usually view it from a very different angle. They tend to say something like the following: 'I don't care what you call it or how you define it. What I want to know is how you deal with it?'. Therefore a teacher's definition will tend to be concerned not with causes but effects and how these effects may be countered. The authors are both teachers. We therefore want to address the question 'How can we help?' rather than 'Why is there a problem?'. Obviously the two are linked but as teachers we are happy to leave research into causes to those who have skills in identifying them. Therefore the definition of dyslexia we have chosen concentrates on how the condition affects a child's learning. It is based on the one used in the Special Needs Code of Practice (see Chapter 8):

A Definition of Specific Learning Difficulties (Dyslexia)

Children who have difficulties in reading, writing, spelling or manipulating number, which are not typical of their general level of performance. They may gain some skills in some subjects quickly and demonstrate a high level of ability orally, yet may encounter sustained difficulty in gaining literacy or numeracy skills. Such children can become severely frustrated and may also have emotional and/or behavioural difficulties.

How Can Dyslexia be Identified?

Many booklets and leaflets on the subject provide the reader with a checklist of dyslexia indicators. We are going to provide you with one but be warned, such checklists can be misleading. Giving an anxious parent such a checklist can be a little like providing a hypochondriac with a medical dictionary. It is sometimes difficult not to fear the worst when faced with such information. It is very human to react like a famous river boatsman, when faced with a dose of flu and a medical dictionary:

> I remember going to the British Museum one day to look up the treatment for some slight ailment of which I had a touch. Hay fever I fancy it was. I got down the book and read all I came to read and then in an unthinking moment I idly turned the leaves and began to study diseases generally. I forget which was the first distemper I plunged into, some fearful devastating scourge I know. Before I had glanced halfway down the list of symptoms it was borne in upon me that I had fairly got it. I sat for a while frozen with horror and then in the listlessness of despair I again turned over the pages. I came to Typhoid Fever, read the symptoms and discovered that I had Typhoid Fever. Must have had it for months without knowing it. Wondered what else I had got. I turned up St Vitus dance. Found, as I expected, that I had that too. I began to get interested in my case and determined to sift it to the bottom. So I started alphabetically. I looked up Ague and learned that I was sickening for it and that the acute stage would commence in about another fortnight. Bright's Disease I was relieved to find I had only in a modified form and so far as that was concerned I might live for years. Cholera I had with severe complications. Diphtheria I seemed to have been born with. I plodded conscientiously through the twenty six letters and the only malady I could conclude I had not got was Housemaid's Knee.

Three Men in a Boat, Jerome K. Jerome

So our checklist is going to be very brief. It only contains three elements and it comes with a health warning: the danger is that you may see in the child's behaviour what you expect to see or what you fear to see, and not what is actually there.

For instance, many checklists will say that a child's reversing of letters or words is a dyslexic indicator. Well, it can be. What they often fail to add, however, is that reversing letters is common before the age of seven. What they actually mean is that if a child persistently reverses letters throughout his/her writing and not just occasionally confuses a 'b' with 'd' or a 'p' with a 'q' (which is normal for a young child), then dyslexia could be indicated. We are thinking of the kind of checklist which you will see pinned up on the library or supermarket noticeboard among the Neighbourhood Watch leaflets and advertisements for Line Dancing classes:

IS YOUR CHILD DYSLEXIC?

it might say, and then will continue:

DOES HE OR SHE WRITE LETTERS BACK TO FRONT?
IS HE OR SHE BEHIND THE REST OF HIS/HER CLASS IN READING?
DOES HE OR SHE FORGET THINGS?

and so on. Such notices will often ask if the child has difficulty remembering things like telephone numbers or multiplication tables. They may not add that most children, with no learning difficulties at all, will forget these things sometimes, will mix up their times tables occasionally or forget something as soon as it is told to them. They do not say that one of the frequently noted characteristics of some extremely bright children, who have no learning difficulties at all, is a tendency to be disorganised and absent-minded. What matters more with all these factors is their severity and how often and how persistently they occur.

More important than all these factors individually is the child's overall pattern of learning. Children can learn to read and write very well if their only problem is a tendency to write some letters and words backwards. In the long term they will almost certainly naturally mature out of doing so. If they have a short-term memory problem which is uncomplicated by other factors, then they can be readily shown how to compensate for this with simple and effective memorising strategies. If their only difficulty is in concentrating on their work, then the teacher should be able to help them overcome this problem with relative ease. If, however, they seem capable in other ways but have contrasting difficulties with reading or spelling; if they persistently and very frequently write words and letters backwards; if they always forget things as soon as they have heard them; if they seem hopelessly unable to concentrate or pay attention to their work; then you can begin to feel justified in sensing they have a significant problem.

So treat our checklist, which follows on p.6, with the same degree of caution that we have advised you to treat any others. If you are a teacher, check your views out with home. If you are a parent, discuss your responses with school. If you are unsure how to interpret it, get hold of someone with training and experience in assessing children with special needs. In the UK, the special education section of your Local Education Authority would be very willing to advise you on this.

CHECKLIST
for possible dyslexic difficulties for child aged 7–11

(A)   Firstly, the child must have a difficulty with
basic literacy or numeracy skills

Where the child has difficulty	*Example*
Difficulty in reading	Did not achieve Level 2 in the UK national tests at the end of Year 2
	Cannot read at all or hardly at all
	Reading is clearly behind most other children in the class
	Reading age is very low compared to own age
Difficulty in spelling	Did not achieve Level 2 in the UK Year 2 national tests
	Cannot spell simple regular words like 'hat' or 'dogs' or 'chip' or 'home'
	Cannot spell name
	Spelling age is very low compared to own age
Difficulty with number	Did not achieve Level 2 in UK national tests at end of Year 2
	Cannot do simple addition or subtraction sums
	If they are taught, has great difficulty in remembering multiplication tables
	Number age is very low compared to own age
Difficulty with forming handwriting	Handwriting is clumsy and badly formed
	Handwriting is very immature
	Handwriting is illegible or barely legible

Secondly, these difficulties should be specific.

(B)   If he or she does have these difficulties, do they seem out of place with
his or her ability in other areas of the curriculum?

Kind of underachievement	*Example*
The child seems to be orally brighter than his/her reading, writing and number skills seem to show	In the UK, achieving Level 3 in Speaking and Listening at the end Year 2 but only getting Level 1 in Reading or Mathematics.
	Comments from the teacher such as: 'I am really surprised he has difficulty with reading. He seems so bright when he answers questions in class.'
	'The child is nine and has a reading age or spelling below 7 years but seems orally at least as able as his or her peers.'

Kind of achievement	Example
The child has a specific difficulty with one aspect of English or Mathematics	In the UK, getting Level 3 in reading, but Level 1 in spelling or handwriting.
	Comments from the teacher like: 'He can read back to me what he has written and it sounds good, but I cannot read it at all' or 'The content of his written work is excellent but its full of spelling errors'
Major differences between his/her ability in some subjects compared to others	In the UK achieving Level 4 in Science at the end of Year 2 but only Level 1 in English.

Thirdly, other factors may apply.

(C)   The child may also have one or more of a number of other difficulties or indicators which are often associated with dyslexia

Difficulty or sign	Example
The child has difficulty in concentrating or attending.	He or she often daydreams or seems inattentive when they should be working or listening
The child becomes easily confused between left and right	The child will have great difficulty in explaining to you how to find a particular place i.e. for the older child, you are taking him or her to a friend's house in the car and s/he keeps misdirecting you
The child seems very clumsy	Cannot tie shoe-laces very well or had greater than normal difficulty in tying them
	Drops things more than the average child or trips over things or walks into them more than is usual
Quickly forgets things	Reads a word at the top of the page but then cannot read it, or misreads it, further down the page
	Keeps forgetting regular school activities, like swimming or taking dinner money
	Forgets messages
	Forgets arrangements
Has difficulty finding the right word	Often struggles to find the right word when talking to you. It is on the tip of his/her tongue and it stays there
Has difficulty in remembering things in the correct sequence	For the older child this would include getting telephone numbers mixed up, or getting the wrong order of words when spelling
	Often mispronounces longer words; gets the syllables mixed or in the wrong order or leaves them out

continued on next page

Difficulty or sign	Example
Others in the family have had similar problems	There appears to be strong evidence that dyslexia can run in families. At the time of writing some British researchers believe they may have discovered a *'dyslexic gene'*. They believe they have proved that dyslexia can be inherited. By the time you read this it may be established fact — or another team of researchers may have proved them wrong!

It is the cluster of difficulties and their severity which are the important factors. It is the picture of the child as a whole which matters. If the child is or appears to be struggling with reading or writing or numbers at school and seems to fit the general picture found in the checklist, then parents and teachers need to have a serious discussion about this. If the child appears to be intelligent but to be significantly underachieving in reading, writing or numeracy, then discuss it together, decide if there is a problem and the strategy to adopt to overcome it. Get more information. Involve the School's Special Needs Coordinator. If you are the Coordinator but need advice, ask the educational psychologist or a specialist teacher from the LEA. You will also find a list of resources and useful addresses at the end of this book.

What are the Main Effects of Dyslexia on Children's Learning?

Our definition of dyslexia was more concerned with effects than causes: the effects of dyslexia on a child's ability to learn efficiently in school. This section outlines those effects. The key word in the definition is 'specific'. A dyslexic child's difficulties will tend to be focused within a small part of the curriculum. The problem is that this small part is often central to the child's ability to cope effectively elsewhere. If a child's specific difficulties were an inability to read French then only performance in that subject would be affected. If a child cannot saw wood accurately there will be problems in making a coffee table but Science or Geography will not suffer. If, however, they have major reading or spelling difficulties, or their handwriting is illegible or their organisations skills are weak, then their work in virtually all subjects could be severely affected. In this sense the description 'specific' is misleading. *The difficulties may be specific but their effects are general.* This is why dyslexia can be so disabling to the child in school. The chart on p.9 summarises the areas mainly affected by dyslexia. Fuller details can be found in the next seven chapters.

The effects of specific learning difficulties (dyslexia) on a child's ability to learn

Primary Effects

Reading	The ability to read is vital to nearly all areas of the curriculum. Poor reading skills inhibit independent learning, deny the child access to the 'other worlds' of books and can seriously undermine self esteem and self confidence.
Spelling	Often in the long term poor spelling is a greater problem than poor reading. It will severely restrict children's ability to show what they know in class and in examination settings it may lead to inappropriately low marking and underrating of work.
Writing	The major difficulty here is an obvious discrepancy between children's ability to show their thoughts and knowledge orally and in extended writing. Many dyslexic difficulties come together to adversely affect writing.
Handwriting	There are three main factors here: legibility, speed/fluency of writing and maturity of style. Deficiencies in any area can seriously affect children's ability to perform effectively in class. Some children have deep seated specific difficulties with handwriting itself (dysgraphia).
Number	Nearly all dyslexic children will have similar problems in number to those for literacy, e.g. reading the text and correctly writing the shape, direction and sequence of numbers. Some children have deep seated specific difficulties with number itself (dyscalculia).

Secondary Effects

Organisation	Organising time, space and sequence are the major difficulties here. Examples are bringing the right equipment to school on the right day, keeping to the timetable and homework.
Attention/ Concentration	Another difficulty which extends across the curriculum and which can severely undermine progress.
Language	Typical problems here are putting thought into words, difficulties with naming things, remembering the sequence of syllables when saying long words. Often called the hidden handicap, its effect can extend across the curriculum.
Memory	This difficulty tends to underlie all the others. It is as much a cause of writing difficulties as it is of remembering which day of the week PE kit is needed or the next bit of that mental arithmetic problem.
Emotional/ Behavioural	These difficulties are more an effect than a cause. Low achievement leads to low self esteem and frustration which lead to poor behaviour which leads to lower achievement, lower esteem, worse behaviour in a declining spiral.

Dyslexic Pupils Have Problems With More Than Reading

Dyslexia is more than just a difficulty with reading. There are many bright dys-lexics, especially older children, who are adequate or good readers. However, these pupils will still have some very specific and often quite severe difficulties with other tasks across the curriculum. Dyslexia literally means a difficulty with words. It comes from the Greek:

DYS = DIFFICULTY

LEXIA = WORDS

That a child has difficulties with words means more than just problems with reading. It can also mean difficulty with a number of related skills which are described in the next few pages.

Difficulty in matching the correct sound with the correct written symbol

In books or in reports on children you may see this referred to as sound–symbol correspondence. This means correctly matching the sound a letter makes with its written form. Difficulties with this skill can cause unforeseen problems.

When reading, children have to find the word in their head which matches the written symbol they see on the page in front of them. By written symbol we mean a letter, a word or part of a word or a number. This is not always as easy as it may seem. For instance, many dyslexic children have difficulty in reading words which look and sound like each other. They will often read one of these pairs of words as though it was the other. Look at the following **pairs of words which are easily con-fused with each other**:

was/saw

were/where

house/horse

who/how

Do these kinds of confusion seem familiar? When children confuse the words in these pairs, they have difficulty in matching the word to the symbol because both words seem so alike to them. This is often irritating for parents and teachers because the words concerned are usually very common and they seem simple to read. Remember though that many young learners may also make these same kinds of confusion. If the child is very young it may be something that he or she will mature out of naturally.

It might help you to understand the problems dyslexic children have here if you think of the difficulty most adults have when trying to identify identical twins. We can become very confused between them, even when we know both twins very well. Their similarities confuse us and prevent us spotting quickly the very slight differences which should allow us to distinguish between them. This is exactly the kind of difficulty facing dyslexic children when they come across similar-looking words. If they persistently make this kind of mistake, encourage them to think about what the words mean. Usually the sense will give them a clue as to which word is right in context, as the following examples show:

Example: Distinguishing between visually similar words

'The Robinson family lived in the *house* at the bottom of the garden.'

If children here read 'house' as 'horse' then they are not reading for meaning. They should be able to work out that the word is 'house' from its context. People do not live in horses!

I *saw* the man *was* a very good runner.

Here again children should not confuse these two words, 'was' and 'saw', because their meaning is so different. If children do make this kind of error, they may be over-reliant on using the shape of words to work them out, rather than using their meaning.

When spelling, the child has to match the sound with the written symbol. This is more difficult than reading because the sense of the passage being read does not help with the spelling. To learn to spell effectively, the dyslexic child needs to be taught very carefully the rules which underlie the matching of sound to symbol.

Naming ability: finding the right word at the right time

This section concerns a difficulty some children have with finding the right words at the right time. We all have this problem to some extent, but for many dyslexic children it is a major difficulty. In reports it may be referred to as an **expressive language difficulty**.

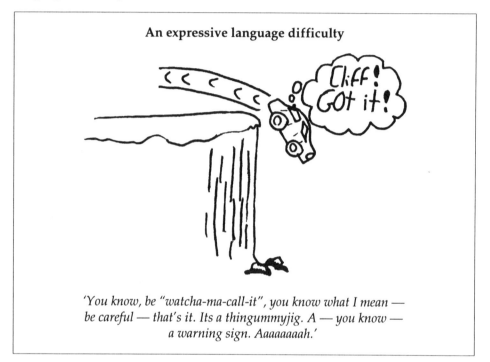

An expressive language difficulty

*'You know, be "watcha-ma-call-it", you know what I mean —
be careful — that's it. Its a thingummyjig. A — you know —
a warning sign. Aaaaaaaah.'*

Is this familiar? Is the child sometimes accused of not seeming bothered about giving oral answers in class or of being tongue-tied? If so it could be related to a dyslexic-type difficulty.

Understanding what other people say

The ability to fully understand what is being said to you is fundamental to learning. Problems with it are often referred to as being a **receptive language difficulty**. Many dyslexic pupils experience such difficulties.

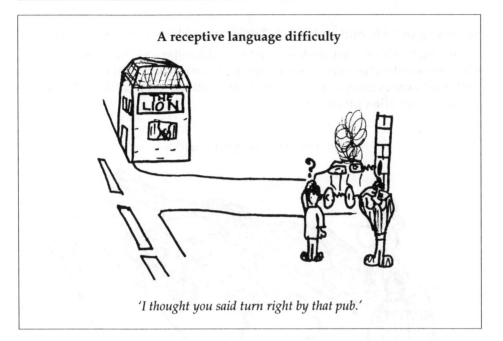

A receptive language difficulty

'I thought you said turn right by that pub.'

Not being able to remember and recall information

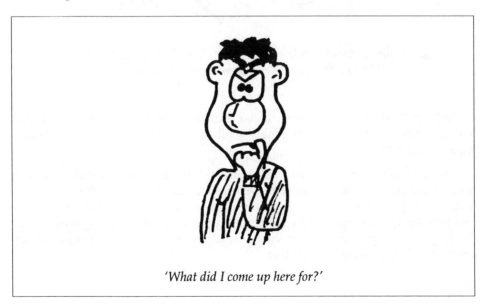

'What did I come up here for?'

Processing quickly and accurately information which is in the memory

A difficult skill for many dyslexic children is the ability to hold several pieces of information in their heads at the same time, and then be able to extract the one piece of information they need from all the others, at exactly the the right time. This ability is called **information processing**.

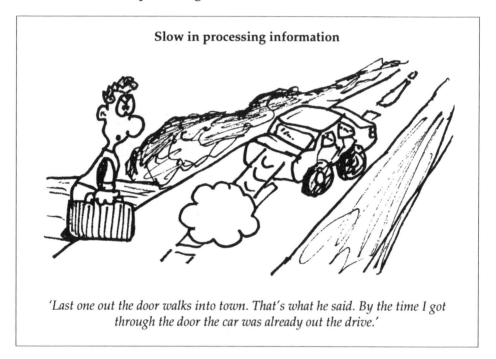

Slow in processing information

'Last one out the door walks into town. That's what he said. By the time I got through the door the car was already out the drive.'

Dyslexic children may have particular difficulties here when they are under pressure: whether the pressure is danger of missing a train or the fear of not finishing an exam in time.

Dyslexic children are therefore likely to have difficulty at school with a number of skills and concepts other than those involved in reading. It is vital that parents, teachers and peers know this and are aware of the implications. If the effects of these problems are ignored, the child's ability to learn may be seriously impaired. Effective support for dyslexic children should be about the whole child, not just about improving their reading and spelling.

A Guide to Using This Book

Chapters 2 to 7 deal with specific areas of learning which may be affected by dyslexia. They range from reading to study skills, to the consequences of dyslexia on subjects across the curriculum. Each chapter starts with the main effects of dyslexia on that area of learning. It then describes ways in which the child may be assisted to overcome or compensate for those effects. The emphasis here is on ways in which the parent or non-specialist teacher may help. Chapter 7 contains a section on understanding the jargon commonly used in assessment reports.

Chapters 8 and 9 are concerned with the legal and semi-legal processes which have been developed for children with special educational needs including dyslexic children. The Code of Practice for Children with Special Needs is described and analysed in detail. The Code is a vital development in England and Wales. It lays down the procedures and practices which should be adopted or emulated by schools and Local Education Authorities. It emphasises school and parental rights and responsibilities. The statementing procedure is covered in depth. *Chapter 10* is a review of the kinds and forms of support which exist for dyslexic pupils across the country.

A Final Word looks at dyslexia from a completely different perspective. It argues that being dyslexic may not be wholly to children's disadvantage. It comes close to saying that being dyslexic can be a good thing, something to be celebrated not regretted. It argues that as communication and development systems become ever more sophisticated, through advances in information technology, so dyslexic people's strengths will be increasingly emphasised and their weaknesses minimised. To give you a taste of this: it is already possible for one machine to write the words which someone speaks into it and for another to read aloud the pages it scans. Calculators will continue to do the calculating. Soon it may not matter that dyslexics struggle with reading, writing and basic calculation. If they are freed from their inhibitions in these areas, are future dyslexics poised to follow their illustrious predecessors, like Einstein and Leonardo Da Vinci, and make a major contribution to the world, via their enhanced skills of creative thinking, invention and innovation? This chapter speculates that they might.

At the end of the book, the reader will find a series of useful appendices: a glossary, lists of further reading, resources and useful addresses.

Summary of Chapter 1

This chapter

- outlined the main aims of the book;

- defined what we mean by dyslexia;

- described how dyslexia can be identified;

- described the main effects of dyslexia on children's learning;

- showed that dyslexia is more than a problem with reading.

Chapter 2

Reading

This chapter looks at how children learn to read. It is a complex area. Different 'experts' have different ideas about the reading process. We have tried to concentrate on those areas where there is most agreement but have included some ideas which would not usually find their way into a book on dyslexia. We start by generally describing key aspects of the reading process and then consider some useful methods which will help dyslexic children become more fluent and able readers.

The Dyslexia Continuum

Dyslexia can be far more than a difficulty with reading. Although reading difficulties are experienced by most dyslexic children at some stage, most eventually learn to read adequately. Some have only minor problems with reading. Others have very significant and prolonged difficulties. It is important to understand that different children are affected to different degrees by the condition. Dyslexia should be thought of as a continuum of need from a very minor difficulty to a very severe one, with many different levels in between. The main stages of this continuum are shown in the following diagram:

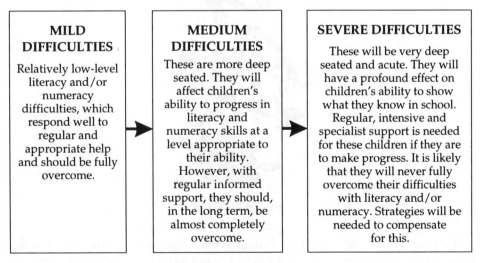

MILD DIFFICULTIES	MEDIUM DIFFICULTIES	SEVERE DIFFICULTIES
Relatively low-level literacy and/or numeracy difficulties, which respond well to regular and appropriate help and should be fully overcome.	These are more deep seated. They will affect children's ability to progress in literacy and numeracy skills at a level appropriate to their ability. However, with regular informed support, they should, in the long term, be almost completely overcome.	These will be very deep seated and acute. They will have a profound effect on children's ability to show what they know in school. Regular, intensive and specialist support is needed for these children if they are to make progress. It is likely that they will never fully overcome their difficulties with literacy and/or numeracy. Strategies will be needed to compensate for this.

A dyslexia continuum

Being at the wrong end of this continuum is not a recipe for despair. The most severely affected children may never be able to read fluently and independently. However, they can become adequate readers, able to extract the information they need from text and to read for pleasure.

We say this confidently because experience shows that even children with the most severe difficulties will respond to systematic, appropriate, structured, cumulative and multi-sensory teaching of reading. This chapter explains what this teaching involves.

The Consequences of Being a Non-reader

The ability to read is vital: it gives children independence and a sense of belonging to, and identifying with, their own society. Being able to read means belonging to the club: the world of writing and all that involves. Society places great value on the ability to read. In most cultures it is seen as a basic human right. Non-readers can feel excluded, frustrated and isolated if they are denied it. In a literate society they may feel like outcasts whose worth as a citizen is undermined by their inability to make rapid sense of those black marks on the page. An English reader can gain an insight into this feeling of futility by attempting to read a word derived from a completely different writing system. The Chinese system is a case in point. It uses pictograms of a word to express its meaning. Here is an example:

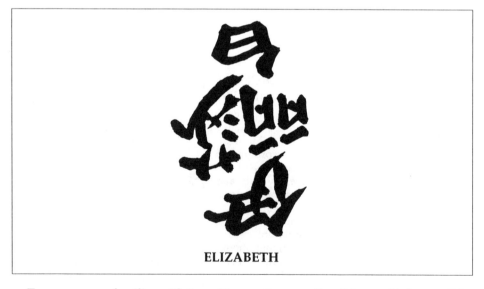

ELIZABETH

To someone unfamiliar with its writing system, reading this word is impossible. It is a meaningless collection of symbols which, without a key to interpret them, are unreadable. Not knowing how the symbol can be read as 'Elizabeth', it could literally stand for anything in the universe. This is how non-readers see writing in their own language. Even though they can speak and understand it, its coded form, its written form, remains a closed book to them. Unable to unlock the code, it is alien and indecipherable.

Some Thoughts on Reading Ages

Before we go any further we want to raise the issue of *'reading ages'*. These scores can be a source of great concern to both parents and teachers. However, they are often given more weight and value than they actually deserve .

A reading age is a rough measure of children's reading ability compared to the average for their age. It is a very simple in concept. The average 7-year-old child is expected to have a reading age of 7 years; the average 11-year-old, a reading age of 11 and so on.

Reading ages are obtained by giving the child a standardised reading test. The word 'standardised' means that the test has been piloted with a large number of children. From the scores of these children on the test, an average score is calculated for each age group. Put very simply, the average score for all the 7 year olds taking the pilot test might be 20. In the resulting reading test children will have to score 20 to obtain a reading age of 7.

Reading ages are useful when trying to estimate the severity of children's difficulties. The teacher can, by considering how far below the average for their age children are, estimate the kind and amount of extra help they will need. These scores are often used by Local Education Authorities in assessing whether or not a child needs a statement of special educational need (see Chapter 9). However, we would strongly advise you to treat all such scores, including spelling ages, number ages and comprehension ages with caution. They are only an estimate of children's ability on a single test at one moment in time. Children might come up with a very different result, if they had used a different test on a different day. This is especially the case for dyslexic children. A test administered by someone known and liked by the child, in a familiar place, at a time when the child is feeling fresh, is likely to give a higher reading age than the same test given by a stranger in a strange place last thing on a Friday afternoon. So treat any test scores with a healthy scepticism. They will give you a rough idea but no more than that. Given that 'health warning' we list here **some examples of reading ages and what they mean**. In doing this we are trying to show you the kinds of reading skill which need to be acquired to register the age concerned.

A rough guide to what reading ages mean

Reading age	Reading skills usually developed by this age
Under 7	Children are building up basic reading skills. They are likely to following a reading scheme or graded 'real-books' programme at school with both phonics and look/say methods also being used.
7–8	Basic reading skills are still developing. Children will enjoy reading a relatively simple text supplemented with many illustrations. There will still be a tendency to read word by word.
8–9	Children are gaining in experience and growing in confidence. Longer, more complex books are chosen and there is less reliance on picture cues than before. This is a time of consolidation.
9–10	The mechanics of reading are largely mastered. Reading is being used confidently in other subjects across the curriculum. Children can read silently for pleasure and extract information from simple reference books. Being read to is still enjoyed.
10–12	They are now confident and independent readers, able to cope with nearly all the reading encountered across the curriculum.
12+	Children are now fluent and accomplished readers, confident in tackling a range of texts. Reading style is automatically adapted to suit the reading purpose.

What is Reading?

Superficially, reading is no more than a 'de-coding' skill. Words are made up of a code called letters. These letters correspond to the sounds of spoken words. As we read we hear the sounds of the words in our heads. To crack the code we need to know which sounds correspond to which written letters. Simple. But it is both harder and easier than this to read. It is harder because sounds made by the letters are not always consistent. It is easier because the reader does not have to rely on the sounds alone in a word to be able to read it. The following subsection contains a little sequence which we have based on the work of a writer on reading called Jeff Hynds. It should help you to see what we mean when we say that reading involves more than just linking letters to sounds.

The reading process

You think you can read? Then read this:

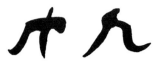

'That is cheating', you will say. I meant, read something written in our alphabet. Fine, read this:

nach quch qab qogh burgh

You know all the letters. Why can't you read it? You will naturally reply that we are still not playing the game. You meant read something that was written in your own language or another language with which you are familiar. (If you are a Star Trek fan you may have recognised the Klingon for various body parts.) Here is our next example:

the aerobic composting of separately collected putrescible household waste via a dedicated kerbside collection system from households and the creation of a useable product.

In one sense you can read all the words. They are written in your own language. But, like us, I expect you do not *fully* understand what they saying. In that sense you cannot read them. Reading is about understanding what is written. Computers have been trained to read text which is entered into their memory. But they cannot actually read those words in the sense of understanding what they mean. Reading is about getting meaning from text. Quite often you do not even need to know the sounds the letters make to read a word. Look at the next examples. We have taken some key words out. See if you can read those missing words:

. . . was Queen of England in 1997.

He . . . the meal in the microwave oven.

The . . . to Malaga from Heathrow took three hours.

If you got the words right — and we know you did — then you can sometimes read without even seeing the words involved. So reading is not only about learning sounds. It is also about using your brain and your experience of the world to work words out from their context. You know that microwave ovens cook food. Obviously you take flights from airports. If you live in Britain you know who the monarch is and so on. So you could immediately read the words involved even though they were not there! The important point is that dyslexic children should be encouraged to read like this, should be praised for using their brains and their knowledge of the world and their language when tackling difficult words. They must not always rely on phonics. In our examples 'flight' and 'Elizabeth' are quite hard to read from their sounds alone, but very easy to read from their context. We accept that there is a major place for phonics teaching in the reading process, but only as part of a broad and balanced reading programme.

Reading Cues

The ability to read without always having to 'work the word out' using letter sounds, brings us to heart of the reading process. When we read, we can use several cues to help us with words that we do not immediately recognise. These cues are used simultaneously in order to read successfully and automatically. The table lists eight important reading cues:

Reading cues

Reading cue	Example	Explanation
The pictures on the page	The text says: 'The elephant picked up the log.' The picture is of the same thing.	The picture will often help the child with a new or difficult word.
The shape of the word	i.e. crocodile, television	The child becomes used to associating the shape of a familiar word with the word itself.
The sounds made by the letters	'Put out your hand to s-t-o-p the bus.'	Some words can be worked out simply by sounding out their letters. These letter sounds are phonic cues.
Knowing words by sight	e.g. 'the, to, is, was, when, where, what, there, their, who, why'	Some words occur so often that it is worth children learning them by heart as 'sight words'. Thirty-two words make up 50% of all children's reading.
The context of the word	'When Jim got home he switched on the . . . to watch the News.'	Providing you have the necessary knowledge, sometimes the context can give you the word without you being able to even see it. These cues are also known as semantic cues.
Grammatical rules	When Jim got home he . . . on the television to watch the News.	The English writing rule that a verb follows the noun means that the unrecognised word must be a verb or doing word. These are also known as syntactic cues.
The initial letter of the word	'Manchester C . . . won the League.'	At other times the context will only give one of several options. For these words a quick check of the initial letter sound will often give the correct word.

Reading cue	Example	Explanation
Several cues working together	From an article on recent successes for Wales: 'The North Wales team W beat West Ham in the fifth round of the FA Cup.'	For the reader who does not come from Wrexham or is not a keen football fan, the first letter clue combined with the context of a known result might not be enough for them to crack the code here. However, the added context of the result being part of a feature about Wales might just tip the balance.

Happy Learners are Successful Learners

Most accomplished readers do not remember how or when they learnt to read. It just seemed to happen naturally and easily. They appear to have learnt how to use the reading cues almost automatically, with as little effort as they learnt to speak. They do not appear to have had to go through the difficult, laborious process that some others have experienced.

There is a further effect of this. Those who learnt to read quickly and easily tend to associate reading with pleasure; those who struggled, with frustration and failure. If children are struggling to learn, they are likely to be experiencing these same feelings. How this is handled is very important.

Parents and teachers can themselves become anxious when children are not reading as well as their peers. That anxiety can communicate itself to the children and increase their growing feelings of insecurity and self-doubt. This, in turn, will impede their progress further. A downward spiral can quickly develop, where anxiety leads to increased failure, which causes greater anxiety which, in turn, impedes progress further and so on, until the child virtually gives up: you cannot fail if you do not try. So the main message is this:

HAPPY LEARNERS ARE SUCCESSFUL LEARNERS

How often have you heard a sports commentator say something like: 'He's beginning to relax now and play his natural game and he's so much the better for it'? Children learning to read are no different. Some of the techniques we will talk about later in this chapter are mainly designed to help children relax and enjoy the learning process so much, that they forget they are learning.

People tend to worry most when they have not got the information they need to fully understand what is happening. Patients talk about the relief of finding out what is wrong with them, even when it is something very serious. In the same way, parents and teachers of struggling children are often relieved when they are told that the children are dyslexic. 'At least we know what is wrong. Now we know we can try and do something about it' is a common reaction.

Children too can respond very positively when told they are experiencing dyslexia. We are wary of labelling people with disabilities by referring to them by the name of their disability. Therefore, we talk of children with a hearing impairment not 'deaf' children, of children with a physical disability not 'handicapped' children. Often the children themselves reject such niceties, happily stating they are deaf or handicapped. This can be true also of children with dyslexia, because it is usually seen, by those who understand its meaning, as a positive label. This is because identifying children as being dyslexic means that we know how to help them and can be sure that the help will be effective.

For this reason, the main carers in the lives of these children should remember that dyslexia is a positive concept. They need to have the maxim — 'happy learners are successful learners' — firmly imprinted on their minds. Some of the fears parents have if their children are struggling with reading are shown in the illustration on the opposite page. It is our intention that this book should provide answers to each of the questions posed.

Many parents of struggling readers have self-doubts and queries like this. Many teachers have them also. It would very easy to rephrase each question so that it came from a teacher not a parent. They are genuine questions. They should always be taken seriously. They need to be answered. The remainder of this chapter attempts to answer them by explaining the different ways children learn to read and the stages they normally go through to become readers. It looks at what can be expected at each stage. It shows how, in partnership, parents and teachers can help children become fluent readers.

The Essentials of a Reading Programme

Key elements in a reading programme for children with moderate and severe specific learning difficulties

The programme will be systematic, appropriate, structured, cumulative, thorough and multi-sensory:

- **Systematic**: the programme will be devised and followed consistently.

- **Appropriate**: the programme will be at a level consistent with children's needs and will aim to interest and involve them.

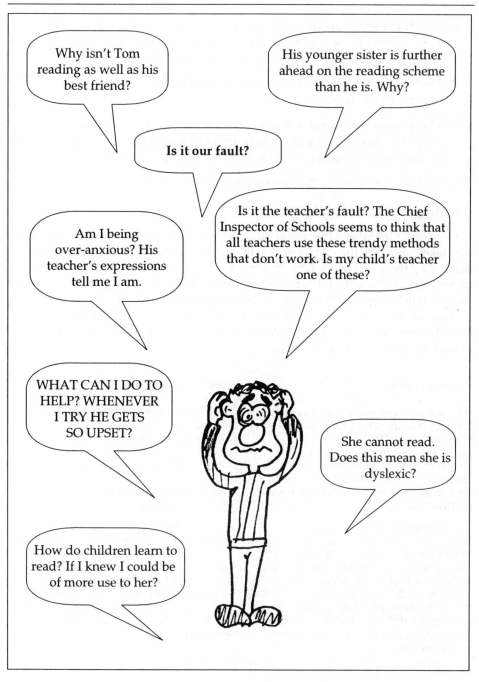

- **Structured and cumulative**: the programme will be built upon a sound framework involving the children learning from a series of small, finely graded steps. Previous work will be continually revisited and reinforced.

- **Thorough**: each element in the programme will be covered in sufficient depth to allow its full mastery.

- **Multi-sensory**: the programme will use methods which use as many senses as possible: vision, hearing and touch. This will include **'saying'**, not a sense as such but an important part of the multi-sensory programme.

These elements are considered in detail later in this chapter.

The Stages of Learning to Read

One way of looking at the reading process is to think of it as a journey. This journey takes children through a series of broad stages in learning. In the table illustrating these stages, we have linked them with those that a learner driver also passes through. We hope this will help you understand the reading process and also show you that there is nothing mysterious about learning to read. It is as simple, or as difficult, as learning to drive a car. (We have adapted this chart from one presented to a recent British Dyslexia Association Conference by Bernadette McClean of the Helen Arkel Centre in London.)

Learning to drive	*Learning to read*
(1) Many people, before they ever sit behind a steering wheel, think that learning to drive is easy. This is a popular misconception, especially with 17-year-olds. At this stage, before they have tried to learn, learner drivers do not know what they cannot do. They are **'unconsciously unable to drive'**.	(1) Initially young children will have no idea that they cannot read. They do not know what they cannot do. They may enjoy books, like handling them, looking at the pictures and being read to, but they will not realise that the marks on the page have a meaning. In one sense they are **'unconsciously non-readers'**.
(2) When they take their first tentative lesson on the road, they suddenly discover that driving is not easy. They get in, switch on and the car lurches down the road and stalls. Coordinating the brake, clutch and accelerator while you change gear, watching the other traffic and thinking where you are heading is a difficult set of skills. They are now at the stage of being **'consciously unable to drive'**.	(2) When they start to learn to read, they will begin to understand that the marks are the same as the words they speak. They realise that they have a meaning. However, they will not know how to reach the meaning from the marks. They know what they want to do, but they have not yet learnt how to do it. They are **'consciously non-readers'**.

Learning to drive	Learning to read
(3) They persevere and practice all these new skills. Their driving becomes smoother and more controlled. They still have difficulty coordinating the more complex manoeuvres. They need to concentrate very hard to achieve what for the experienced driver are simple tasks. Their driving skills are not automatic. They know what they have to do, but are not assured in doing it. They are **'consciously able to drive'**.	(3) They practice. They are read to, they read along with a better reader, they start to use the reading cues we described earlier. They link particular letters with particular sounds, they use the pictures, the overall sense of the story or sentence. They are beginning to become readers. But they still have to concentrate hard and read word by word. What they do not know is getting less and less. They are **'consciously literate'**.
(4) After much practice and experience, well after they have passed their test, they become skilled drivers. They can drive smoothly and do not have to think about basic driving skills like engaging the clutch before selecting the gear. It is now an automatic skill. They have become **'unconsciously able to drive'**.	(4) When they reach the final stage, they emerge as fluent and independent readers. They read automatically without having to consciously think of the cues involved. They read with pleasure, able to concentrate wholly on the what the words mean rather than how they sound. They are now **'unconsciously literate'**.

Reading is Easy

Reading can be made to seem a very difficult task. From one perspective, it appears to be such a complex skill that it is amazing anyone actually learns to do it. It seems impossible to know and to do simultaneously all the things required to read fluently. This is deceptive. We perform many more complex actions routinely. Nearly everyone can speak without even thinking about how they do so. But consider the simultaneous skills needed for speech:

Speaking is easy? Some of the skills necessary for fluent speech

- Be able to control your breathing to force air over the larynx.

- Be able to use the muscles of the throat and mouth to form the sounds.

- Know where to put your tongue for different sounds.

- Know which shape to make with your mouth for different sounds.

- Know how loud you want to make each sound and how to achieve that volume.

- Decide how you are going to say it: crossly, pleasantly, firmly, politely, sarcastically, wisely, sadly, happily, sceptically, hopefully.

- Choose the right words to convey your meaning.

- Know the meaning of all the words you use.

- Know the sounds of all the words you use.

- Put the words in the right order.

- Understand what is said to you in reply.

- Work out your response.

- Keep an eye on the kids playing on the road and an ear ready for an expected phone call.

How do we learn to apply all that knowledge and those skills simultaneously? It seems impossible. Yet the reality is that many 3-year-old toddlers do it routinely and have quite complex conversations. Skill for skill, silent reading is much easier than speaking but most children arrive at school able to speak well enough to make themselves understood. So we should not exaggerate the complexity of reading. It is less complex than many other skills which we all develop as a matter of course. It begs the question: if this is the case, why are there so many children who struggle to read and so comparatively few who struggle to speak? Maybe it is because most children learn to speak with the close attention of their parents, while most children have to learn to read in large, busy classrooms. Maybe it has something to do with the way they are taught. That is what we are going to consider now.

Different Views of the Reading Process

The idea that reading is comparatively easy is not a view shared by all reading experts. Some of these people see reading as a highly complicated skill, whose mastery places great demands on teacher and learner. You will probably have heard that there is no universal agreement about how children learn to read. This is as confusing for teachers as it is for parents. There are many different views of the reading process, but two main schools of thought predominate: the phonic method and the psycholinguistic or real-book method. It is on these that we are going to concentrate.

The phonic view

From the phonic perspective, reading is a building-up process. Words are made of letters. Letters have sounds. Each sound is called a phoneme. There is a set of rules for combining the phonemes into words. Children learn the phonemes and the rules for their combination. Then with practice they can build up any word they encounter.

Learning to read with phonics

At first children learn the individual phonemes or sounds:

a b c d e f g h i j k l m n o p q r s t u v w x y z

They then learn how to combine these sounds to make simple words.

b + a + g = bag

r + u + n = run

Then they learn that some letters combine to make a single sound

s + h makes the combined sound **'sh'**

Then they learn to add this combined sound to other letters to make more complex words:

sh + o + p = shop

or

p + o + sh = posh

Gradually, more sound combinations are added to increase children's ability to build up more and more complex words.

hat

hats

hatch

hatches

hatching

hatcher

thatcher

nuthatch

nuthatches

That is the theory. What could be more simple or logical? But reality is more complex. There are 26 letters in the English alphabet. These letters, either singly or in combination, make approximately 44 sounds. Eighty per cent of English words are phonetically regular. For these words, the method works very well. However, we cannot avoid the major problem in phonics tuition which is those other 20% of words which are not regular. The next section gives some examples of the phonic variations present in many English words.

Phonic variations

Let us start with the famous 'cat'. No problems here. Children learn the sounds made by the individual letters 'c-a-t' and then, when they are blended together, there it is: 'cat'. Nothing could be easier. So with 'chat'. The child is taught the sound of 'ch' and once again the letters fit smoothly together to make the word. But what about 'Christmas'. The 'ch' is not behaving as it did in 'chat'. It is not making that nice, soft sound any more. This 'ch' sounds more like a 'k'. Going by its sounds, 'Christmas' could be quite logically spelled as 'Kristmas'. Many young spellers do exactly that. Perhaps this word is an exception? But there are very many exceptions in English. Think of the combination of letters: 'ough'. It can make eight different sounds. Here they are:

tough bough through ought thorough cough dough hiccough

'ough' is an example of the same letter combination having eight different sounds. On other occasions the reverse happens; when different letters or letter combinations make the same sound. In the following example, eight different letters or letter combinations make the same vowel sound 'a'. Note the sound of the underlined letter/letters:

able came rain hay grey weigh great

Then there are silent letters. This is a little confusing for children. First they are taught that letters correspond to sounds and you put the sounds together to make words. Then they are told that some letters make different sounds in some words, then that some letters in some words do not have a sound at all. Here are some examples of the latter. There are many more. The silent letters are underlined.

gnat know mate pneumatic thumb

There are logical, linguistic reasons for these inconsistencies. These can be taught to children. For instance the 'ch' in Christmas is of Greek origin. Using phonic methods children will be given examples of other words in which 'ch' makes the same sound (a list of these words may be found on p.36). Teaching them in this way will assist the child to learn them.

However, it cannot be denied that phonic instruction would be more effective without these inconsistencies. They undermine the *exclusive* use of phonics as a means of learning to read. This is not to condemn the system. It is an essential element of any programme for dyslexic children. The ability to use phonic knowledge, to break words down into their component parts as well as to build them up to their whole, helps develop skills which are vital to children's overall ability to become fluent readers. Children need a core of phonic knowledge to be able to read but they need much more than phonics to become fluent readers. Many experts have led savage attacks on the use of phonic instruction, often by pointing out the kind of inconsistencies highlighted here. Usually these attacks are very selective, as illustrated in the evidence they choose to criticise the method. What must be remembered is that much of the English phonic system is regular in nature. Once a working knowledge of this system has been mastered by children it will prove an invaluable aid to them in the early stages of reading. The relevance of intensive phonic instruction is, to some extent, dependent on where children are placed on the dyslexic continuum. Children with mild difficulties will probably need very little more phonic tuition than their fluently reading peers. More severely dyslexic children require much more than this. They need an in-depth understanding of the phonic system and how it works in relation to the English spelling system. The further along the dyslexic continuum children are placed, the greater will be the part played by phonics in their reading programme.

The psycholinguistic view

This approach attracts much publicity. It is often called the 'real-book' method. You may have heard it being blamed in the press for alleged poor reading standards in our schools. Yet the method has a great deal of logic. Its basis is that children should be encouraged to read naturally in the same way that they learnt to speak naturally.

Children learn to speak for many reasons:

- Because they want to. They quickly learn that if they say 'Mum' after their Mum says it to them, then they get a nice hug and Mum looks very pleased and gives them a reward.

- Because they are surrounded by other people speaking. They learn to speak by hearing them and imitating them.

- Because they are encouraged to. For instance, by being helped on the spot if they make a mistake. Jane says: 'I want a pollilop.' Dad does not say 'Don't be so silly. Its a lollipop. Don't you know anything?' He says: 'It's lollipop, love. Lollipop. You want a lollipop. Lollipop. You say it. Lollipop.' Jane says 'Lollipop'. Dad says 'Fantastic. Do you want a green one or red one?' This child was given a quick lesson on the spot about the correct pronunciation of the word and was then immediately rewarded with what she wanted when she got it right. She soon got the idea that this speaking business is worth getting right.

Psycholinguists believe that children learn to read most readily when their experiences of reading most closely resemble the way they learnt to speak. (They believe much more than this, but it is near to the essence of their theories.) To encourage children to want to read psycholinguists believe that children should learn with the very best of children's books: the ones with the most attractive pictures, the most vivid language and the most exciting or interesting stories. They believe that children should learn to read by reading with other more accomplished readers, in the same way that they learnt to speak by listening and responding to more skilful speakers. So they encourage extensive reading practice at school and especially at home. They do not dismiss the importance of children knowing their phonic sounds but they do not believe that having these skills alone enables children to become skilled and enthusiastic readers.

Where Does It Leave Us If the Experts Do Not Agree?

You should not become too worried about this lack of agreement. We believe that teachers may teach differently according to which set of beliefs they accept, but if they use those methods consistently, flexibly and conscientiously then their pupils will tend to learn well whatever system they use. Just as two different gardeners may grow leeks in completely different conditions, with completely different fertilisers and varieties of seed and yet both produce prize-winning exhibits, so two different teachers can help two different groups of children to become equally successful readers using wholly different methods of teaching.

In our experience, very few teachers use one or other method exclusively. They let the experts carry on arguing with each other from their opposite viewpoints and take from each what they feel to be the best ideas and practices. In other words they use a variety of methods. In line with the psycholinguistic school they will select books for children which have the most attractive illustrations, the most exciting language and the most engaging storylines. They will encourage parents to read often at home with their children and also to keep on reading to them. However, they will also make sure the children have a core of sight words, know their letter sounds and how to use a variety of methods to help them work out difficult words.

The scope of this book does not allow us to go into any depth on the theory behind learning to read. We have concentrated on describing some generally accepted methods of teaching and learning reading. We have concentrated on those methods which are used for dyslexic children.

The Skills and Knowledge Necessary for Effective Reading

As we have stated, there are many **different methods of teaching reading**. These are the main ones:

- whole-word recognition methods,

- phonic instruction,

- reading schemes linked to either or both of these methods, using children's literature not reading schemes,

- paired reading,

- apprentice reading.

In the latter two methods the learning reader develops his/her skill by reading with or alongside a more skilled reader.

We do not believe that there is a definitive method to teach reading. As we have said there is much ideological debate favouring different methods but in our experience most teachers take the sensible middle course and use a mix of methods. The late Jean Augur, a past Education Director of the British Dyslexia Association, stated that children fall into four categories of learning readers:

How Children Respond to Reading Methods

(1) Those who learn to read by any method.

(2) Those who, with time, adapt to any method used.

(3) Those who survive in spite of the method used.

(4) Those who fail because of the method used.

Notice she does not 'blame' the child in any of these categories. She does not, for instance, say:

- Those who fail because they are not interested.

- Those who fail because they are of low intelligence

- Those who fail because they are dyslexic.

She is not saying either that there are no children who are unmotivated or of low intelligence or dyslexic. She is saying that children who fit these descriptions may need teaching in a different way, if they are to learn to read successfully. Unmotivated children need encouragement and reward. Children of low ability need very structured, programmes which build knowledge up in small steps. Dyslexic children need — well, we are coming to that. The message is that no child deliberately sets out to fail at reading. That may be what they say but it is not what they mean. The other message is that many poorly motivated or low ability or dyslexic children learn to read very well indeed. The difference between them and their similar peers who are not learning probably lies within factors such as the quality of teaching, the size of their classes and how home supports them. In other words, the difference lies in factors over which the children have no control: how they are being taught and how their parents help them.

Children have different strengths and weaknesses. As a consequence they learn in different ways. It is important that their reading programme reflects these differences. In particular it is vital that their learning to read is not dependent on one exclusive method of teaching. The danger is obvious. If some methods of teaching suit some children better than others, then if only one exclusive teaching method is chosen, it will inevitably not be the best one for every child in the class. There is a useful adage here which might make the point just as well:

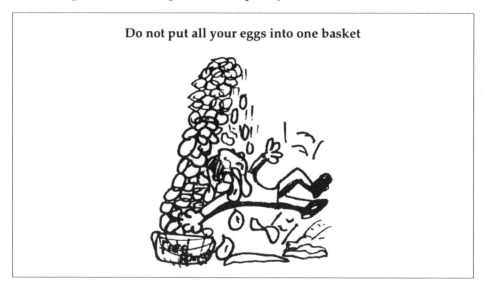

Do not put all your eggs into one basket

In the following pages we give an overview of a variety of different methods for teaching reading. In doing so we reinforce our belief that parents and teachers should be familiar with a range of methods; that all methods should be available simultaneously in the same classroom, with different emphases for different children depending on their underlying strengths and weaknesses as learners. We would be surprised — despite the myths promoted by the media and politicians — if you could find many teachers who do not already teach in this way.

Whole word recognition

This method is often referred to as 'Look and Say'. It is best suited to children whose visual skills are stronger than their hearing or listening skills (their *aural* skills). It works on the basis that immediately the child sees the word, they should be able to read it. There is no need to think about it or 'work it out'. See it and say it. Some teachers refer to words learnt in this way as a child's 'sight vocabulary'. As we have said before, some children are primarily visual readers and some primarily aural readers. This method is most effective for the visual reader, for the child who can remember the shape of words better than their sounds.

High frequency words

Many specialist reading teachers who work with struggling readers try to build up in each pupil's mind a sight vocabulary of the most commonly used words in English writing. There are different versions of which words these are. A popular list with many teachers is the McNally/Murray list of high-frequency words (the first 100 words are given in the table).

The McNally and Murray key words

in	was	I	he	is
it	a	the	that	to
and	of	are	for	you
had	so	have	said	as
not	they	with	one	we
on	his	at	him	all
but	old	be	up	do
can	me	came	my	new
get	she	here	has	her
will	an	no	or	now
did	by	if	go	down
just	out	your	into	our
went	them	well	there	were
big	call	back	been	come
from	only	first	off	over
must	make	more	made	much
look	little	some	like	right
then	their	when	this	two
see	about	could	before	other
which	what	where	who	want

The main aim in teaching these words is that children will be able to recognise them instantly. If they learn them all, then in theory they will be able to immediately read a large percentage of all the words they encounter in books, magazines and newspapers. In these circumstances it seems worthwhile spending some time learning them. This is especially the case when you consider that a large number of these words are not regular phonically. A quick and certain knowledge of how these words are spelt is also useful in helping children build up simple sentences.

Family groups of words

It is not only high-frequency words which are taught in this way. Children may be taught naturally forming groups of words which contain the same cluster of letters. Here are some examples:

Example: 'ch' saying 'k', Greek in origin

Christ   Christmas   Christian   Christopher

chemist   chemistry   chemical   chorus   choir

chronicle   school   stomach   ache   echo

orchestra   technical   mechanical   architect

architecture   anchor

Example: 'que' saying 'k', French in origin

unique   antique   oblique   cheque

picturesque   grotesque   discotheque

Example: Use 'ck' after a short vowel sound

knock   back   lick   peck   stick   duck

struck   stack   pick   click   clock   cluck

Example: 'nk' at the end of words

bank   bunk   clank   clunk   dank

dunk   thank   stank   think   blink

wink   plank

In this way, children's phonic programmes are reinforced by their look/say programme and vice versa. Teaching children these family groups of words helps to fix them in children's minds visually and aurally. You need also to refer to the section in Chapter 3 on 'Onset and Rime' (see p.73), a new way of looking at phonics.

Grouping words specific to a subject

Some secondary-school teachers encourage children to learn key words in a particular subject's vocabulary. This can be of great benefit to them, especially if the
specialist teacher links with the subject teacher and teaches important new vocabulary just before they come up in the lesson. An example is given for geography but
similar lists can be drawn up for any subject:

Example: Geography

climate   coast   terrain   weather   Ordnance Survey   Australia   Venezuela

economics   chalkface   limestone   meandering   erosion   ecology   Africa

To help children learn them more efficiently, these words should, wherever possible, be grouped according to common letter patterns.

The vocabulary in a reading-scheme book

Some early-years teachers teach children the vocabulary of a reading book in this
way before they are given the book itself to read. By ensuring that the book can
therefore be read with little difficulty, children are given a strongly motivating
sense of achievement and confidence..

Methods of teaching whole-word recognition

A common method is to use flashcards. The mere mention of flashcards will
cause some teachers to flare up in indignation. A typical comment might be: 'Flashcards are boring. Meaningless. They will put them off reading for life.' There is no
doubt that their incorrect use can have this effect. However, used sensitively and
with variety and humour, they can help some children, by providing them with a
secure base which instils confidence to try for themselves later.

When using flashcards, children are initially given the word to look at, usually
written on a card, where possible with a visual clue to its meaning on the reverse.
They are then asked to commit that word to memory, trying to remember the visual
image of the whole word shape. Multi-sensory learning is essential here for dyslexic
children. They must say it as they see it, as they hear it and as they touch it.

Dyslexic children will need considerable overlearning on each word.
'*Overlearning*' means that they are encouraged to remember it on many occasions
in a variety of settings. This will help to fix it in their minds. Children who are
having difficulty with reading need to have the word so firmly imprinted that it will
not only stay in the mind but it can be easily recalled when the word is encountered
in print. So they must practice the words in one setting, recall them in another, get
them in a game the next day, practice them with Dad the same night, play a

computer game with them the day after and so on until they stick. Once they have stuck, the conscientious teacher will return to them at regular intervals to reinforce and revise them.

Problems can occur with this method when words have the same or similar shapes. For example, the words 'horse' and 'house' are easily misread or mistaken for one another.

When dyslexic children mix up visually similar words, the teacher will always try to point out a logical reason to help them distinguish between them. Going back to our example, if they confuse 'horse' and 'house', the teacher may draw them back to the meaning of those words. It is quite difficult to think of examples where the words 'house' and 'horse' can be easily interchanged in terms of meaning. Have a look at these sentences and you will see what we mean:

I rode my *house* to Calvary Cross.

He had to fit a new drainage system to his *horse*.

Children should easily be able to distinguish between them when they concentrate on their meaning not their appearance.

An alternative method is to find internal clues in the words to help children remember the difference between their letters. One way with the above pair of words would be to point out to them that the word 'horse' has a rider in it — 'r' — and 'house' does not. This helps to cement the difference between the words in their minds. It is better to stress, explain and concentrate on only one of the confused words. Give them a firm grip on that one before moving to the other. Sometimes children have a problem in remembering any detail of a word besides its shape. The word that they read has no resemblance, except in shape, to the actual reading of the word. These children are relying entirely on word shape as the cue to reading it. The frequency of reading a word correctly using only this technique is not high.

Children need to learn these words in a variety of settings. Boredom and anxiety must be kept to a minimum. They can practice by using simple games like these:

- Large flashcards with the words in coloured letters to point out the different letters in the word.

- Pictures with clues on them — as funny or quirky as possible — to help children remember.

- Snap cards making sure the words are read and checked by the children.

- Flashcard games

- Making the word to be read more tactile (touchable). Paste the letters and shake sand on them. Or use wooden and plastic letters.

- Matching the same word in a game with you. The winner reads the word (a form of Pelmanism).

- Word bingo

- Writing the word on children's backs, on the back of their arms, in the sand, feeling the word in sandpaper.

There is much the parent or teacher can do with such games to help children learn to read without them being aware that they are being taught. This will help them to see that reading is for pleasure, something they can associate with success not failure. Failure breeds more failure.

As adults we can often avoid doing the things we do not like. If we hate gardening, we can go golfing. If we hate washing up, we can buy a dishwasher. If we are poor writers, we can take a job which does not require writing. Children do not have that choice. They cannot successfully get through school unable to read or write. If they are poor at these skills, school will constantly remind them of their failure. If they are struggling then you will need to bolster their confidence, give them success and encouragement with these simple activities. A little and often is recommended. If children get upset then do not blame them. Think about changing your approach. Many successful teachers have a belief which goes something like this:

If the child is not learning, change the teaching.

This is especially true of learning to read. As we stated earlier, children have different learning styles. It is important that their learning to read is not dependent on one exclusive method. The danger is that a single chosen method will not suit the learning style of all the children in the class. For instance, if children have difficulty in remembering the shapes of word, then learning through the 'Look and Say' method will be counter-productive. There is a technical term for this weakness in remembering whole word shapes and a poor memory for letters. The term is *'dyseidetic'*. Dyseidetic children will have difficulty in building up a stock of sight words through 'Look and Say' methods. This does not mean they will never learn to read, but that they are unlikely to do so unless they are taught using complementary methods such as the phonic methods which are now considered.

Phonic methods

These methods are in widespread use in the teaching of dyslexic children. Most training courses for teachers of dyslexics place a heavy emphasis on phonic instruction. It is the cornerstone of many multi-sensory teaching programmes, designed specifically for these children. While phonics may be the cornerstone of most specialist dyslexic teachers' stock of methods, its use will usually be complemented with many other techniques and materials. In particular, the phonic programme should be complemented by the use of stimulating, attractive books read with an accomplished reader. This will emphasise that words have meanings as well as sounds, and encourage children to think about and enjoy what they are reading, without constant recourse to 'sounding out' problem words as their only strategy.

What is phonics teaching?

At its simplest it is instructing children in the correspondence between letters and sounds. Here is the content of a **typical multi-sensory phonics programme** designed to help severely dyslexic pupils:

- Letters have sounds as well as names.

- These sounds correspond to letters.

- Letters form two groups: vowels and consonants.

- There are five main vowels.

- The difference between long and short vowels (e.g. between the 'a' sounds in 'hat' and 'hate').

- Long vowels say their names.

- Short vowels say their sounds.

- The importance of the letter 'y' and its uses.

- Some double consonants can be blended together with the sound of both letters heard (e.g. bl, st, tr). These are called 'blends'.

- Some triple consonants can be blended together with each of their sounds heard (e.g. spl, scr, shr). These are also called blends.

- That 'q' and 'u' work together to make a multiple sound.

- That some letters can sometimes be silent.

- That when some consonants come together they make a different speech sound to the one you would imagine, (e.g. ch, sh, th, wh, ph). These are called consonant digraphs.

For each of these elements, the important connection between the sound and the letter is made when children read. The teacher must make a judgement as to how extensive the phonic component of a particular child's reading programme should be. At its most comprehensive, a phonic programme is a significant chunk of learning for a child. The table on this page and the chart on the next are illustrations of a full phonic programme which might be offered to a severely dyslexic secondary-age child, whose learning style favours this method. It is important to stress that children offered this programme are not taught these rules in isolation. They are instructed in them in the context of the way in which our language works and is structured. The new material to be learnt is given a meaning and context and is not simply rote learning. Children are treated as intelligent learners of the language. They are given reasons for the ways in which letters and words behave. If they complete the whole course they will have a working knowledge of linguistics as well as being able to read.

A Phonic Programme Order of Work

1. Introduction: terms such as vowel, consonant and syllable
2. Short vowel sounds
3. Long vowel sounds
4. Diacritical dictionary marks
5. Syllable, closed syllable, open syllable and their vowel sounds
6. Consonant digraphs: as ch, sh, th, wh, ph
7. Initial blends: bl. cl, fl, gl, pl, sl, br, cr, dr, fr, gr, pr, tr, str, spr, scr, sw
8. Final blends: nt, st, ng, mp, nd, nk
9. Techniques for learning spelling: NLP and SOS
10. Sounds of y
11. Silent e
12. The use of mnemonics as an aid
13. Murmuring vowels: ar, er, ir, or, ur (er/ir/ur), (ea/ee) (separated for teaching)
14. The long sound of the letters a, e, i, o, u
15. Doubling rule
16. ed endings
17. Vowel digraphs
18. dge, tch, ck after short vowels
19. Diphthongs
20. The sounds of c
21. Plurals
22. The sound of j
23. The sounds of g
24. c/le words — stable final syllables
25. Roots of words.
26. Suffixes
27. Prefixes
28. The six types of syllable
29. Syllable division
30. Word derivations

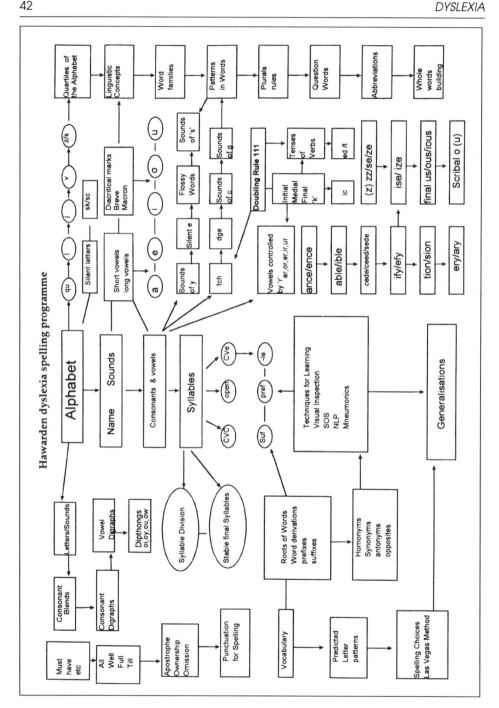

Hawarden dyslexia spelling programme

Just as there are some children who have difficulty learning with whole words (dyseidetics), so there are others who have do not learn well using the phonic method. These children are called '*dysphonetics*'. They tend to be weak at being able to perceive words in terms of their 'sounds' and will try to entirely rely on the 'Look and Say' method. They will usually have a poor memory for sounds (*auditory memory*) and will have problems breaking down words into chunks or syllables. For instance, they may have a difficulty in hearing that 'cat' is made up of three separate sounds. To teach dysphonetic children entirely through a phonic approach would be as counter-productive for them as teaching dyseidetic children through 'Look and Say' methods. However, it would be wrong not to offer both kinds of learner both methods. It would not be wise to put 'all our eggs in one basket'. Multi-sensory phonic teaching will be the core curriculum for most dyslexic pupils, run in parallel with a variety of other learning experiences for the child. However, for dysphonetic children the reverse will apply. Visual programmes will form the core, with other methods complementing it.

Multi-sensory phonic teaching programmes

Multi-sensory teaching means exactly what its name suggests: helping children to learn by using more than one sense. For instance, children can learn the letters in a word by looking at their shape (visual), by feeling their shape (tactile) or by hearing the sounds they make (aural). In other words they can use three senses — sight, touch and hearing — to fix the identity of the letters and word in their memory. Some children learn better visually, some aurally. The idea is, that if they learn new knowledge using all three senses then it is more likely to remain in their memory. Although not a sense, saying is included as a further element in the multi-sensory programme. Thus children hear, as they see, as they touch, as they say.

Some multi-sensory programmes have been specifically designed for dyslexic children. They are the 'hear it', 'say it', 'see it' and 'write it' programmes based on the **British Dyslexia Association guidelines**:

Guidelines for Structured Multi-Sensory Programmes issued by the British Dyslexia Association

- **Phonic**   Teaching is based on the concept that sounds correspond to symbols, beginning with the alphabet and building up.

- **Structured**   Teaching is organised so that each part is an integral piece of a jigsaw which forms the whole programme. It is structured so that each piece relates to the others in an organised and planned way.

- **Sequential**   Teaching is progressive and builds up in a planned and organised way. It is like building a house. The foundations must be secure before the walls can be erected, the walls before the roof. One step follows another in sequence.

- **Cumulative** Teaching should consolidate and build on previous learning in a ladder type progression. Each step is an extension of previous work.

- **Thorough** Teaching is based on the premise that each step of learning must be understood and transferred by the child to general classroom use before going on to the next step.

- **Multi-sensory** Teaching should involve all the senses which can be used in learning to read: hearing, seeing and feeling (saying).

There are many multi-sensory teaching programmes available for teachers. They share the same characteristics: they are phonic based, structured, sequential, cumulative, thorough and involve the use of more than one sense. Typical examples of effective and proven multi-sensory teaching programmes are:

Example A   Teaching Reading Through Spelling (TRTS), Kingston programme and the Hickey Multi-Sensory Language Course

Both these systems use packs of cards which reinforce the teaching of a particular sound to its symbol. The cards give children an opportunity to practice sounds in a multi-sensory way, with the aim that eventually they will automatically link each sound with its symbol. They are probably most effective with primary aged pupils.

Example B   The Personal Phonic Reference Dictionary

At the secondary stage, if children have already been taught extensively using the former systems, then it is advisable to switch to a new one, such as the phonic reference dictionary which is an integral part of the Bangor Dyslexic Teaching System (see recommended booklist). Using this system children complete a dictionary in which they record and illustrate spelling principles and other information concerned with language. The dictionary is their personal property and they are responsible for recording accurately all the elements of their programme within it. This gives them direct responsibility for their own learning. The illustration on the next page is a sample page taken from a secondary dyslexic's dictionary.

3

ă	ĕ	ĭ	ŏ	ŭ
cat	bet	sit	dog	dug
sand	set	sid	frog	hug
stand	lct	bit	cog	mug
band	beg	hit	fog	drug
man	log	mit	dot	bug
brand	left	hid	not	tug
hat	get	mid	bot	slug
bat	stem	hid	cot	
sat	egg	mill	lot	
		hill		

Consonant digraph sh, ch, th, wh

cash	mesh	fish	short	hush
chat	chess	chip	chop	such
that	them	thin	moth	thumb
wham		which		

Consonant Blends: (beginning)

strand	stem	spill	spot	spun
chat	step			drum
pram	dregs			
clam				

Teachers of dyslexic pupils often maintain their own phonic reference book, which can be as valuable to them as the equivalent dictionary is to the child. It can be used as a work of reference, a handbook and a resource book. The following is an example taken from one of the author's personal reference books:

---

ea

(1) This is the second choice for the long 'e' sound when found in the middle of one syllable words.

(2) Many words concerned with eating have a long 'e' spelled that way:

eat   tea   bean   cream   meat   veal   pea   yeast   feast   meal   wheat

(3) Words that are spelled with 'ea' are usually the 'other spelling' of ee:

meat — meet   beech — beach

bean — been   read — reed

peal — peel   seam — seem

Example C   Alpha to Omega

This well known programme has been extensively tried and tested. It is subtitled the 'A–Z of Teaching Reading, Writing and Spelling'. It is written as a manual for teachers and has linked boxes of cards and graded workbooks (see the Booklist for details).

Example D   Onset and Rime

The Onset and Rime technique is very simple and effective. Children are taught to read and spell a frequently used rime, such as 'old' or 'end'. Once this is learnt, they are shown the rime in other words: 'bold, cold, fold, gold, hold, sold and told'. They very soon learn to spot the rime they have learnt, add it to the initial sound, and write or read the whole word correctly.

This technique is explained more fully on p.73.

Psycholinguistic methods — 'real-books'

'Look and Say' and 'Phonics' are an essential part of a child's reading programme. But they are not — or should not be — the whole part of that programme. Think about what you as an experienced reader do when you encounter a new, difficult word. We probably used such a word earlier in this chapter, when we wrote about 'dyseidetic' readers.

Dyseidetic is not a common word. If you learnt it you would probably be one of a tiny minority of people in the country who know what it means. What was your response when you 'read' that word? Did you immediately start to sound it out or were you able to form an aural or sound picture of it in your head straightaway? Are you sure that you have read it correctly? What sound did you give to 'ei'? Are you certain you are right? Of one thing you can be sure. If our explanation was good enough then you will know what the word means and in that sense you can read it. You can see that cluster of letters and give them their correct meaning.

Going back to what we said before, what if you had mechanically misread the word? Using ordinary phonic rules, for instance, what did you make of that tricky 'ei' sound? There are several alternatives ways of pronouncing this vowel sound:

It could be the sound it makes in any of these words: their, seize, reins, foreign, sleight. In fact it is the final sound, the long 'i' sound which is correct. If you did not get this sound right, did you actually read the word correctly or not? In one sense, you did not. The sound you linked to the symbol 'ei' was incorrect. You would have pronounced the word incorrectly. In another sense though you would have read it very well indeed because you fully understood the word's meaning. Which is most important? To pronounce it with absolute precision or to say it with a minor error but fully understand its meaning? We would say the latter. Understanding what you read is vital, absolutely correct pronunciation is desirable.

The core of the psycholinguistic method is that reading is about getting to the meaning of the text in front of you. Consider some English people who have lived in Wales for many years. They cannot speak the Welsh language but, through often hearing it and seeing it, have learnt its basic pronunciation. They could, with a struggle, read a piece of simple Welsh prose well enough for a Welsh speaker to understand it. In one sense therefore, they can read simple Welsh. But if you believe that the real purpose of reading is to understand what you read, to extract the correct meaning from it, then they cannot read it all.

A problem with reading programmes which over-emphasise the visual and aural aspects of reading (such as over-use of phonics and Look/Say methods) is that children may grow to think of reading as a purely mechanical exercise. They will see it as being simply a means of linking letters and words to their correct sounds. They will be concentrating on getting the pronunciation right. The meaning of the word is secondary and if the struggle to pronounce the words correctly is too intense, then the meaning will be lost. This can result in the child 'barking at print'.

Psycholinguists say that children's main aim in reading should be to understand the text. Their most useful asset in this quest for understanding is their knowledge of the world and their knowledge of the context of the words they are reading. Let us assume a six-year-old child is reading the story of the 'Three Little Pigs'. What skills and knowledge does he or she bring to this story?

They will probably know the story well because it would have been read to them before and they will probably have seen and heard it being dramatised on television or on audio tape. They will know certain relevant facts about wolves and pigs, such as pigs do not eat wolves, and wolves are stronger than pigs. They will know that some materials are better for building houses than others. They will know some helpful phonic rules. For example, that word straw' begins with 'str' and the word 'blow' begins with 'bl'. They will know some very common words on sight, such as 'was', 'where', 'there', because they have been taught them.

Here is a typical passage from the story. Let us see what strategies children might use it to read it:

The Three Little Pigs

The first little pig took the <u>straw</u> and built a house with it. Then he sat in his chair feeling *very* pleased with himself. A **knock** came at the door. A deep *voice* said:

'Little pig, little pig, let me *come* in.'

The little pig said:

'Oh no, I will not let you in, by the hair on my <u>chinny-chin-chin</u>.'

The big bad <u>wolf</u> was *angry*. He said:

'<u>Then I'll huff and I'll puff</u> and I'll blow your house down.'

And the big, bad wolf huffed and he puffed and he **blew** the house down.

We have highlighted some of the words in this story to illustrate what we mean. A key to the highlighted words follows.

Form of highlight	Reading cue
<u>underline only</u>	The child will know these words from being familiar with the story.
bold	The child should be able to work these words out from their context.
italic	The child should be able to work these words out using context and the sound made by the initial letter or letters.
<u>italic/underline</u>	The child should know these words on sight (sight-words).

We now look more closely to see how children might have tackled the high-lighted words.

straw	Out of context and with no cues or clues this is quite a difficult word to read. There is that complex string of consonants 'str' blending to make one sound. Then there is fairly advanced vowel digraph 'aw' which cannot be worked out by the sounds of its letters. But children will be familiar with the story before reading it. They will know that the first pig builds a house of straw. They will be expecting the word. They may not get it at first but when they have read on the penny should drop. The word clearly means the stuff the first pig built his house from. The initial letter sound 's' will also help.
very	Again this is quite a difficult to get by phonics alone. The 'e' sound could be short or long and 'y' has many possible sounds. But if the children have been taught the most common sight words then they will know this word immediately without having to build it up from its sounds. Phonic instruction would tell them that next to an 'r' the 'e' is likely to be short and that a 'y' at the end of a word is likely have the long 'e' sound but the child should not need to know this to work it out.
knock	The silent 'k' is followed by the vowel which could be long or short and the consonant digraph 'ck'. In this context there is one obvious word which children can guess at: what do visitors do to doors? They knock at them. Children should then try the word in context. It makes complete sense. Notice too that by solving the word in this way children may well be incidentally learning about that silent 'k' at the beginning and remember it next time.
voice	The main cue for children here is the next word 'said'. What says things and starts with a 'v'? They may well be able to accurately guess 'voice' from this context. Once they have guessed they can check it makes sense: voices do say things and if the speaker cannot be seen then it makes sense to write 'voice' rather than identify the speaker.
come	A tricky little word because the 'o' makes a short 'u' sound when children would expect it say a long 'o' sound. However if they have learnt the most common sight words he or she should read it easily.
chinny-chin-chin	If children knows the story they will know this string of words without needing to sound anything out. If they do attempt to sound it out then almost certainly they are not reading for meaning but relying on their purely mechanical reading skills. They should be encouraged always to read for meaning and use the context to help.
wolf	Another phonically tricky word but they should know it immediately from knowledge of the story plus possibly the first letter clue.
angry	They will know two things about this word. From its context they will know that it describes the state of mind of the wolf. A reasonable guess would that the wolf was upset. Phonically it will be known that the word begins with the short 'a' sound. A word that means 'upset' and starts with 'a': angry!
Then I'll huff and I'll puff	Any child who knows the story will know this sequence of words so well that they will be able to read it immediately because the context tells them what it is.
blew	Children's knowledge of language should help them read this word. The wolf has said he will 'blow' the house down. In this context the word 'blew' is obviously the past tense of 'blow' which they should be able to supply with little difficulty. That is not to say they think 'What is the past tense of "blow"?' They use this knowledge automatically.

What this analysis shows is that the ability to read is more than simply and mechanically translating the squiggles which make up writing into words you can hear in your head. What the children are really doing is translating those squiggles into meaning, into words and sequences of words which mean something.

Although on first sight this seems to make the process more complex, it actually simplifies it. As long as children are familiar with the words they are reading then they can use that familiarity to help them. It is a little like saying 'If they can speak them they can read them'. Of course, it is not as simple as that, but by using their personal experience of language children can predict what may come next. This is an important part of the reading process. Try this out by reading the following:

> As you read this ch . . ., you can use your knowledge of language and your experience of the world to help you guess the word which comes n . . .. This knowledge and ex . . . combined with the first-letter clues should help you work out the correct w . . ..

As skilled readers, we use this type of assisted guessing game all the time to help us read accurately and fluently. Knowledge of the language and knowledge of the world are the key factors. Parents who talk to their children and talk with them, who read stories with them, who enjoy a variety of experiences with them are contributing enormously to their reading and general language development. This can include watching television together, taking out library books or going for walks. It does not have to mean expensive pursuits only available to the favoured few.

Books are best though. **Children learn to read by reading,** just as they learn to walk by walking, to speak by speaking. When children learn to speak they do not practice the small parts of words and then build them up into words. When trying to say 'Daddy', they do not learn the sound 'D' on its own and then add the sound 'a' to make 'Da' and then add the other 'D' to make 'Dad' and then the final 'e' sound to make 'Daddy'. They have a go at the whole thing. They hear Mum saying: 'Daddy's coming home. Daddy is in his car coming home. Do you want to see Daddy! Yes! You want to see Daddy. Daddy! Daddy! Daddy!' Who do you want to see?' The child says: 'Da Da Da'; and Mum says: 'That's right. Daddy!' The child says: 'Da Dad Dad Dad'. Mum says: 'Yes! You said Dad! Wait till he hears you. Daddy. Daddy is coming home.' 'Dad Dad Daddy!!'

The most effective way to learn to read is to read. The more children encounter books the better. There are many ways of **enjoying books**:

- reading to

- reading with

- books as presents

- stories on the television
- stories on the radio
- storyteller sessions at the library
- taped stories
- CD-ROM audio books

Books, especially children's books, can be beautiful, exciting and funny, sometimes all these at the same time. They can — they should — transport the reader to a different world. If the only books children encounter are the mundane and unstimulating reading scheme books used in some schools then they may not realise that reading is such fun, can be so exciting. Few schools will only rely on these books. They will almost certainly make sure that all their pupils have many opportunities to hear the very best of children's books read to them.

That, very oversimplified, is what the real-book movement, which you may have heard so many critical comments about in the press, is all about. To us it has a sensible logic. However, as with Phonic instruction and Look and Say, we do not believe that teaching children via real-book principles alone is sufficient. They also need a core of phonic skills and a stock of immediately recognisable sight-words. The strange thing is we do not know anyone who disagrees with us and we are unaware of any school which rigidly sticks to one system and no other. Yet this seeming myth — that all teachers seem to believe in one method exclusively and in particular that some teachers who believe in real books have been active enough to cause a national decline in reading — thrives in the media and amongst politicians. It is not true. The great majority of teachers use a combination of all the methods we have described in this chapter. As the next section shows, the idea of a national decline in reading standards is itself very dubious. The truth here is vital. If the popular press is right, if reading standards are declining, if teachers are sacrificing their pupils' progress to follow the latest trend, then how can we say so happily that parents should put their trust in these teachers and work closely with them? In reality it is not true that reading standards have fallen. There does appear to have been a minor blip in standards around the time that the National Curriculum was introduced. Apart from that the evidence tends to suggest that standards have hardly changed over the last 40 years.

Is There a Decline in National Reading Standards?

We have discussed an assumed national decline in children's ability to read. All politicians seem to assume this is the case. We are not so sure. There are as many different answers to this question as there are 'experts' who pronounce on it in the papers or on the television. We prefer to leave the final word to the most recent piece of research we could find prior to our book being published. This excerpt is taken from the *Times Educational Supplement* of 11 July 1997.

> 'Reading standards in Britain have remained almost static throughout the past half century, despite the rise and fall of radically different teaching methods throughout that time. Neither the traditional phonics championed in this week's Government White Paper, nor the newer techniques promoted during the past 30 years — and subsequently blamed for falling standards — have significantly improved or worsened average levels of reading.'

This was written by Dr Greg Brooks, Vice President of the United Kingdom Reading Association.

However, Dr Brooks adds that where we are failing is in helping those of our pupils who struggle with reading. He argues that we have in this country a 'trailing edge' of under-achievers. He adds that this is an almost uniquely British problem, not present in other English-speaking countries. 'They don't have a trailing edge. Why should we?' he asks.

That final question is obviously the most important one for readers of this book whose children or pupils may well be members of this trailing edge of under-achievers. In a very real sense dyslexic children are under-achievers: their skills in literacy and/or numeracy are not up to their potential shown in other areas. We believe that if children are identified early enough and helped properly by using a mix of methods matched to each child's specific needs, they should be able to escape from this band of under-achievement.

Paired reading

We will end this chapter with a look at assisted reading methods. These are almost universally acknowledged to be important and successful in bringing on struggling readers. There are many different forms of assisted reading. We shall look at the main one called paired reading. You may not be surprised to learn that it usually involves the assistance of parents. As its name suggests paired reading involves children being directly assisted to read by a more skilled reader.

This technique builds on all three methods described so far: phonics, look–say and psycholinguistics. It helps children learn to read by reading, it encourages them to use phonic and context cues and it relies on their ability to read some words on sight. It pulls it all together. The message for parents is that if your child's school encourages you to read with your child at home, do it, and if they do not, ask them why, and do it anyway . For schools the message is that parents might be your greatest and most under-used resource. They have far more time to read with their child than the busy teacher even if their class has no more than 30 pupils.

Paired reading was devised by an educational psychologist, Dr Roger Morgan, over 20 years ago. It involves children and skilled readers reading the same text at the same time. It is a way of helping at home which will not conflict with the school's teaching, but offers immediate positive support for children's reading. It requires only 5–10 minutes a day. We would advise parents to discuss the technique with their child's teacher or the school Special Needs Coordinator before they use it. Here are the main ground-rules:

(1) *Choosing the book* The children choose the book or reading material they want to read. This can be a little disconcerting when they choose a 'Space Raiders' Comic or an Everton programme rather then the school-reader but persevere. Have faith in their choice. Just like you they are more likely to want to read something they have chosen for themselves. It can help motivate them to read if they feel they are in control of the process. If, however, they have made an unwise choice or they are unhappy with the choice after trying it, do not make them carry on. (Best not to say something like: 'I told you wouldn't enjoy it. Well. Hard luck. You've chosen it now and will have to stick with it.') This is counter-productive. If they are bored with a book allow them to change it, if they want to re-read it, don't interfere. A firm, sensible and consistent approach is recommended. If they want to read a book which is clearly too difficult then agree as long as you are pair reading it with them and can give enough support to make the experience successful and enjoyable.

(2) *Where?* As far as possible you should read together away from other distractions. A comfortable place, away from the television and other children is the ideal. If this is impossible then try and get as near to this as you can. The reading should be undertaken in a relaxed manner with the adult positively wanting to give time to the child. This should give them the message that reading is important — because you are prepared to give time to it, and enjoyable — because you both enjoy it.

(3) *When?* We would recommend once a day for 5 days in a week, for about 5–10 minutes at each session: shorter and it is not worth starting; longer and it can become too much of a commitment for you even if it is not for the children.

(4) *How?*

(A) *Simultaneous reading* The first phase is for simultaneous reading, of reading together as a synchronised pair. The process is very straightforward. Each session begins with the adult and child discussing the chosen reading material, talking about what it is likely to say, the illustrations and so on. At first the adult and child should read simultaneously. You should try and pace your reading to suit that of the child. The idea is to read together in a way which reduces the child's anxiety and increases his or her confidence. The adult acts as a 'scaffold' or prop to the child's reading. The child must read all the words but is not allowed to fail or struggle because the adult is there to immediately supply any words which the child finds difficult.

By reading in this way, children experience, perhaps for the first time, the influence that fluent reading has on meaning. They begin to realise that words, which they have read in the past as separate entities, actually make sense when they are put together. Because they have not got to work so hard on translating the letters into sounds they can concentrate on the meaning of the words. Thus, through this paired-reading activity, they experience an awareness of the importance of understanding what they read. They begin to understand that reading, like speaking is about communicating meanings and intentions to others.

(B) *Towards independence*   As children become more confident in their reading they can move on to the second phase. This is reading alone with close support from the adult for problem words. At this stage the child and the adult agree on a signal which the child can use to indicate that they wish to read alone. The signal can be anything from the child saying 'Now' to a finger lifted to the lips or a gentle nudge in the ribs. When the child gives this signal the adult immediately stops reading and the child continues alone. It is a little like letting go of the saddle of the cycle for the first time or taking the supporting hand away in the swimming pool. It is also like these other situations in that you do not withdraw all help. Just as you run alongside the wobbling cycle or keep you arm just below them in the water so with paired reading you remain ready to help when your child gives the signal. The child signals. You stop reading aloud. The child continues alone. If the child struggles over a word or reads a word incorrectly then you join in again, giving them the correct word and you both continue with paired reading until the child signals again to stop you.

(5)   *Other aspects of paired reading*

(A) *Reading is for meaning*   If children read a word incorrectly but the word makes perfect sense in the passage do not intervene. Reading is about getting the correct meaning from the words. They have done this. If you wish you can always return to the word afterwards and point out that meaning was right but the precise word was wrong.

(B) *Happy learners are the most successful learners*   Paired reading is designed to allow children to practice reading without worrying about the processes involved, to concentrate on extracting the meaning from the words without becoming too caught up in their physical structure. There are not too many rigid rules. It is based on creating low stress, high success and a relaxed and comfortable approach. Too often dyslexic children, for obvious reasons, are very anxious about reading. Parents too, knowing the importance of being able to read, can become very worried and anxious. This anxiety is easily transmitted to children. As a result reading at home can become a traumatic experience.

Tempers can become frayed and the situation can rapidly degenerate to the point where you both hate the experience. Paired reading can help overcome this. It gives instant feedback to the child if an error is made or a difficulty encountered, it reinforces successful reading and discourages children from attention-seeking behaviour or manipulating the situation in order to be noticed. Children can make mistakes without fear of criticism or failure. It is a positive and successful method: 'nothing succeeds like success'. As a result children may begin to feel good about reading.

(C) *Role models*   Paired reading also gives parents the opportunity to demonstrate a role model of what good reading sounds like. How often do we see and hear young children imitating their parents or older relations in their play? It is a recognised way of learning. By reading with children in this way parents will show their children not only how easy reading is but how much they enjoy it. In line with hearing parents read they learn to build feeling, inflection and pace into their reading. For the method to succeed parents and children need determination, encouragement, consistency, books, time, a place and lots of talking.

Purposes for Reading

Fluent readers adapt their style of reading to suit their purpose in reading. If they simply want to extract a piece of information from a reference book, they will scan the text looking for key words until they find what they want. If they are studying a textbook in detail for a examination, they will read every word carefully. If they are reading a thriller, their pace of reading may increase as they reach the climax and so on. This diagram shows the main purposes of reading and the kind of reading which each activity requires.

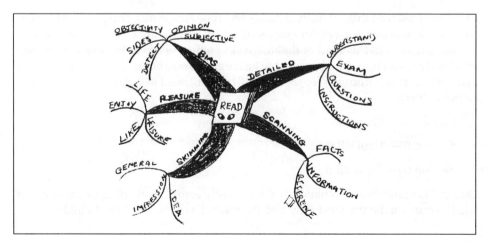

Different types of reading suit different types of purpose. Experienced readers will automatically choose the type of reading which is appropriate to their needs.

Scanning

If readers merely wish to extract a particular piece of information from a text then they will scan it. They do not read every word but hunt for key words which will alert them to focus on that part of the text. Scanning is frequently used to find information from a reference book. It is the most suitable and efficient reading strategy to extract information quickly such as looking for a number in the Telephone Directory.

Skimming

This technique is used when a general impression or overall feeling of a passage is needed. When a passage is skimmed, the reader does not read every word. Instead the reader concentrates on such aspects as titles, headings, words in italic or bold print, diagrams, pictures, key sentences and summaries. These act as clues to give the general impression or feel of a passage.

Reading for accuracy

Sometimes the reader will need to be certain that they have extracted precise information from a text. Following a menu, a guide to a walk or the manual for a construction kit are all examples where the reader must be sure that his or her understanding of a text is accurate. Perhaps of more relevance to dyslexic children is the need to follow examination and test instructions accurately.

Candidates are required to answer Question 1 (Section A) plus one question from each of Sections B and C.

Children must read this carefully if the correct type and number of questions are answered. No marks are given for questions which should not have been answered. Paying attention to this kind of detail is a skill which needs to be deliberately fostered in dyslexic children. They need to be taught how to break down such complex instructions as this into smaller segments. They will need to be taught to write each element down.

Section A — Question 1

Section B — 1 question

Section C — 1 question

Doing this minimises the chance of a very costly error. Misreading or omission of small words can be the most easy and the most disastrous mistake to make.

Many dyslexic children omit small words when reading or even add extra ones. Teaching the ability to read accurately is essential for these children. This is achieved by showing children how to proof-read. To proof-read effectively children must develop the skill to read what is actually on the page not what they think is there. It is an acquired skill and one which improves with practice.

Reading for pleasure

Depending on the nature of the writing, reading for pleasure frequently does not require the reader to read slavishly and accurately every word on the page. There are exceptions to this. The full benefit of a fine poem cannot often be enjoyed without a close attention to the detail of its phrasing. On the other hand, the reader of an exciting 'page turner', which has no pretensions to literature, can merrily race along to reach the final denouement as soon as possible, without worrying too much about reading every word. When enthralled and engrossed in a novel, an avid reader will glide over the words, barely stopping to read them individually.

It is not usually necessary to read every single word on a page in order to understand it. The fluent reader does not look in detail at all the letters of every word but relies unconsciously on clues to predict what is happening. For instance, the upper parts of words and letters are easier to read than the lower ones and the right-hand sides of letters are easier to recognise than the left-hand sides.

The size and shape of the print is important. Writing in block capitals is harder to read than lower case letters:

WRITING IN CAPITAL LETTERS OR BLOCK LETTERS CAN BE MORE DIFFICULT TO READ THAN WRITING IN LOWER CASE LETTERS. WORKSHEETS AT SCHOOL ARE RARELY WRITTEN IN BLOCK LETTERS. BOOKS ARE ALWAYS WRITTEN IN LOWER CASE FOR THE SAME REASON.

As we hope you will appreciate from this book, a page of writing which has text broken up into small paragraphs and which is interspersed with diagrams and pictures will assist the reader to follow and understand the text.

Reading aloud helps children to develop an expression and intonation of speech which is very useful in promoting understanding of the meaning of a passage. A dull, flat, monotone voice is not only boring and uninteresting to listen to, but it can make the meaning boring by association. Actors bring words to life through their intonation and expression. The narrator of a story uses similar skills. Children learn to appreciate the value of this through example. This is why the teacher reading to the class, the parent reading to the child and good quality taped stories are so helpful in developing children's reading.

On the other hand, silent reading can be an equally valuable experience. It is often when the reader is alone with a book or so lost in it that others are not noticed that the real joy of a book emerges. This is when the reader is transported to that other world of books. Dyslexic children, no less than any others, are entitled to this experience of losing themselves in someone else's world.

Stop Press: The Literacy Hour

Since September 1998, most primary schools in England have been expected to spend an hour a day on literacy development. This chapter has frequently referred to approaches to help dyslexic children learn to read, which are different to approaches used for non-dyslexic children. However, there does not need to be a *different* way of teaching dyslexic children to read. Good teaching of reading should be as effective for dyslexic children as it is for all other children. They often need more good teaching than other children, or more of the teacher's time, when reading is being taught. Except for a small number of dyslexic children with deep-seated and intractable difficulties, they do not necessarily need different teaching.

That is what is so exciting and interesting about the Government's ideas for the Literacy Hour. This concept is built on rock-solid effective practice in the teaching of reading. In line with one of the main themes of this chapter, it has not restricted itself to one method of teaching. It has selected the best practice from a range of approaches. It has also 'permitted' schools to put literacy first, to concentrate on getting children literate before other educational objectives. The intense demands on schools to offer the whole of the National Curriculum may have had an effect on their ability to deliver a comprehensive reading programme for all their pupils.

This hour must be devoted exclusively to work on literacy. It cannot be spent, for instance, writing up a science experiment, on the basis that this is also literacy development (even though it is). The Hour must be structured in a certain way. It should provide the following structure for each child in the class:

Structure of the Literacy Hour

The Hour should concentrate on reading instruction. It should provide direct teaching of reading for the whole class or groups, to give every child the best possible opportunities for the following:

- high-quality oral work: discussion, questioning, presentation and reflection;
- carefully guided reading;
- structured teaching of phonics and spelling;
- shared and independent writing.

Every primary class in England will be receiving its hour of direct instruction in reading, every day. Each hour will follow a similar format, a carefully composed mix of whole class and group work, of reading at the level of words and at the level of sentences and passages. A **typical format for the Literacy Hour** follows.

Activity	Group or class	Time/ minutes	Example
Sharing a text together	Class	10–15	The Hour begins with a a whole class teaching session. An enlarged text is used. The teacher model reads the text.
Word/sentence work	Class	10–15	Together, children look at elements of the text, i.e. vocabulary or spelling, depending on the teaching objective for the hour.
Directed activities related to abilities and attainments of the children	Small Group	25–30	Each group works on a set literacy task. Some groups work independently. The teacher concentrates on those groups who need help most.
Review and recap	Class	5–10	The teacher pulls the children together again and they whole class reports back and reflects on the work they have been doing.

In one sense the whole idea of the Literacy Hour is a major experiment. No-one knows for certain if it will significantly raise standards of literacy, to the levels targeted by the Governmenment the year 2001: that 80% of children aged 11 will achieve Level 4 in English. This is a very ambitious target. Whatever its overall effect, the Hour's concentration on structure, on review and recall, on a balanced approach to the reading curriculum and on a significant amount of time being devoted each day to literacy development, should benefit dyslexic children. Even if it does not, of itself, improve the literacy skills of these children, it should raise general levels of achievement and thus free up extra time and resources for dyslexic children, to be taught individually or in small groups. So we thought it would be a good idea to end this chapter by briefly describing the Literacy Hour, and in doing so, convey this simple message.

If all teachers of reading adopt the approaches involved in the Literacy Hour, conscientiously and thoroughly, with all children, then the number of dyslexic children with significant difficulties in reading and spelling should be seen to drop considerably.

Welsh readers should note that the Literacy Hour does not apply in Wales. Instead, a national literacy policy has been adopted, promising many of the same ideas and principles as the English Literacy Hour but with far greater flexibility.

Summary of Chapter 2

This chapter

- showed that dyslexia is experienced on a continuum from mild to severe difficulties;

- described the kinds of skills involved in reading;

- showed that happy learners learn best;

- described different views of the ways in which children learn to read. (whole-word recognition, phonics and psycholingusitics);

- showed what is meant by multi-sensory teaching;

- described the new 'Literacy Hour' concept in the UK.

The chapter contains many examples of simple, easy to use methods to help children become more effective readers.

Chapter 3
Spelling

This chapter is concerned with the spelling skills of dyslexic children. It explains why these children may have serious spelling problems and how those difficulties may be best overcome. First, however, it seeks to show that being dyslexic is not just about reading and spelling: it can affect the whole of a child's life.

Dyslexia and Spelling

Christopher Robin in the Winnie-the-Pooh stories may have been dyslexic without knowing it. Look what he says about his own writing:

> my spelling is wobbly. It's good spelling but it wobbles and the letters get in the wrong place.

His spelling is rather inaccurate and has many of the types of mistake made by dyslexic pupils. Here is another example, on a notice attached to the door of Owl's house:

PLES RING IF AN RNSER IS REQIRD.

PLEZ CNOKE IF AN RNSR IS NOT REQID.

This notice again betrays Christopher Robin as a potential dyslexic speller. Here are some of his **dyslexic-type spelling errors**:

Mistake	*Explanation*
PLES	He has written the letter 'e' as if it is saying the sound of its name. If it did say its name the word would sound right. However, in English spelling, a single 'e' on its own does not have the sound of its name unless it is followed by another 'e': 'be**e**' or 'tre**e**' or 'her**e**' or 'ced**e**'
PLEZ	Here he has spelt 'please' a different wrong way; a common feature of dyslexic spelling.
RNSER	Once again he is confusing the name of the letter — in this case 'R' — with its sound.
CNOKE	Logical?: The 'c' is making a hard sound like a 'K' as it does in 'cot' or 'candy'.

The Connection between Reading and Spelling

An inability to spell accurately may severely affect how the writer is seen by others. For instance, some teachers and parents may associate weak spelling with low intelligence. Poor spellers may make the same assumption about themselves. *'I cannot spell, because I'm thick'* is a familiar defensive refrain from such children.

On first seeing Christopher Robin's notices, we might initially make some very superficial judgements about him based on his spelling. We might assume he was very young and at the beginning stages of learning to write or that he was older but that he had been poorly taught. Looking at that notice again we might find ourselves thinking: *'Not only is his spelling poor, but his reasoning is no better.'* Whereas if his spelling had been immaculate we may have interpreted his apparently silly mistakes about knocking bell-pushes and ringing knockers more generously:

Here is the notice again, this time spelt correctly:

PLEASE RING IF AN ANSWER IS REQUIRED.

PLEASE KNOCK IF AN ANSWER IS NOT REQUIRED.

Now that the misspellings are removed the pleasing irony of the bear's thoughts are much more evident. We are able to pay more attention to the meaning of the words.

We have the same piece of writing with the same meaning. In each case, the meaning is absolutely clear. Yet, because of the difference in spelling, the general abilities of each piece's writer can be viewed in opposite ways. This can also be the case for dyslexic children. Weak spelling can bring continual undervaluing from their peers and teachers and can prevent them from reaching their true educational potential. They lose out twice over. Firstly, the message of their writing is reduced in the eyes of their readers because of their poor spelling. Secondly, because they are afraid of making mistakes, they may not write as fully as they might otherwise have done. They might, for instance, not choose the word they really want because they cannot spell it. They will opt instead for an inferior or blander word because it is within their spelling vocabulary.

Spelling is a cross-curricular skill. If children are only weak in Science or PE or Art then they will only have to live with that weakness when they are actually doing the subject itself. But spelling comes into nearly every subject. Even Art will have calligraphy lessons and just when they think they are safe in PE the rainclouds may erupt and the teacher will suggest writing a story on football instead.

Teachers may unconsciously undervalue a child's work because of its poor spelling. In a written exercise where the main aim is for children to get the content and meaning right, they may be given a lower mark because their spelling was poor, not because they had got the content or meaning wrong. A genuine example of how this may happen follows.

One of the writers once conducted an experiment with a large group of teachers. He divided them into ten sub-groups. He gave five sub-groups a copy of a story written by a dyslexic child in his own handwriting. The story was very good but it had many spelling mistakes and the handwriting was large and immature. The other five sub-groups had a copy of the same story, but this time it had been typed up with all the spelling mistakes corrected. The actual words were exactly the same. Each group was then asked to mark their story. They could give it from a grade one (lowest) to five (highest). They were expressly told ONLY to mark it for the CON-TENT of the story, to ignore the spelling and handwriting.

The five groups with the original, uncorrected story gave it between a one and three grade with most giving a two. The five groups with the typed story gave it at least three with some awarding a five. One of these latter groups said they thought the child would go to university easily with his ability to use language like that.

So spelling matters, but unfortunately spelling problems tend to take longer to correct than those with reading. This is particularly true in the case of bright dyslexic pupils. Good reading ability is not automatically associated with good spelling, but weak reading ability is usually mirrored by poor spelling. In other words, weak spellers who are good readers are rare but good readers who cannot spell are common.

Why is this so? It is because reading and spelling involve different skills. They are independent of each other. Reading is a decoding process. You start with the code on the page, the words. It is a process of recognition based on symbols. The code is in the form of letters and the way those letters are put together to make words. To read those words you need to decode them. To do this you need a key. In reading the key is made up of several cues of clues which the reader may use to crack the code. The table on page 22 in the previous chapter listed these cues, e.g. the pictures on the page, the shape of words, the sounds made by letters, the context of a word. As the next section shows this is not the case with spelling.

The Skills Needed for Good Spelling

Whereas in reading you have to decipher or decode what you can see, spelling is almost the reverse. When spelling you have to encode. This means to put letters together to make the word you can hear or remember seeing or hearing. There are several different ways to **encode**:

Kind of spelling	Example
Hear to write: You hear the word and then write it, working out the sounds which go with the symbols or letters and then changing these into the written word.	Spelling test, dictation passage, writing down homework.
See to write: You see the word and then you write it from memory.	Copying from the blackboard, taking a word from a dictionary.
Remember the image of word to write: Each of us has a memory bank of words which we can spell. The child needs to be able to locate the picture of the word in the mind and then accurately transfer it into writing.	Free writing, essay writing, letter writing, writing a cookery book.

To spell accurately the child needs to be able to:

- hear clearly and be spoken to clearly;

- have a good memory bank of words which he or she can spell and be able to re-trieve those words from the memory;

- remember which letters make which sounds and when;

- remember the order in which the letters should go.

The Role of Speech and Hearing in Spelling

Clear speech and hearing play an important part in ensuring that spelling is accurate. Children must be able to speak the word clearly to be able to spell it. If they say 'somefink' then they will probably spell it that way. When children struggle to spell a difficult or unknown word they will often use a technique known as *'auditory rehearsal'*. This means that they say the word slowly to themselves. As they do this, the word is heard by being spoken internally. 'Speaking it aloud' is a common and useful aid to spelling correctly.

Similarly, if children have problems hearing high-frequency sounds and difficulty in distinguishing between them it is unlikely that they will be able to hear the difference between, for example, 'th' and 'ph' and 'f'. Being able to spell them from just hearing them is even less likely. This is because if children have weak hearing in a sound frequency, then all sounds in that frequency will sound the same. One way for children to overcome this is to encourage them **to 'feel' the difference in the sound**. This can be done in several ways:

- Through the use of a hand-held mirror to see how the mouth forms different shapes for different sounds;

- By showing how the tongue is positioned differently for each sound;

- By letting them feel how air is expelled differently from the mouth.

The ability to feel for the patterning in a word is also important as far as spelling is concerned. This can be done through hand movements when writing with a pen on paper as well as the touch of fingers on a keyboard when word processing. In reports, this skill is referred to as *'kinaesthetic'* ability. Joined up handwriting, or cursive script, is recommended as soon as possible when teaching dyslexic children to write. This is because of the importance of their being able to feel the groups of letters as units in words.

Cursive writing = joined up writing

Words and strings of letters which have a high incidence of coming together in parts of words can then be built up, for example: '-ing', '-ed', '-ight', '-ought' and '-dis'. Cursive writing has the added advantage in that it helps with the left to right movements which are often confused. It also reduces the number of times a letter has to be started. Once mastered, cursive writing improves the speed of handwriting and produces the kind of mature hand which is especially important for children's sense of self-esteem.

As a word is written, the ability to see the difference between say, a 'b' and a 'd', 'm' or 'w' and 'p' and 'q', becomes essential for spelling. Confusion between 'b' and 'd' is common among young children. It is normal. However, if the confusion persists for longer than expected, then the child needs to be taught how to distinguish them. The twin analogy helps here also. You know the names of the twins, but you cannot remember which name goes with which child. It is the same difficulty when similar-looking letters are confused. Children know the name of the letter but cannot remember to which symbol it belongs. The correct link between the picture of the word and its name must first be established in their memory. It must be firmly anchored on a memory 'peg'. Once written, children must be able to check a word by sight and recognise whether it does not look and feel right.

Language skills, such as being able to break words down into chunks and syllables and being able to rhyme, play a useful role in developing spelling skills. Many parents sing or recite nursery rhymes to their young children. These children are likely to learn to read and spell more easily than if they had not had this early experience of rhyme, of the repeating patterns of sounds that some words share. Children seem to have a natural curiosity about words. They experiment with them, play with them, try them out in different situations. Effective parents and teachers build on this natural affinity with language. Dyslexic children will benefit from making this natural process more explicit. Collecting patterns of words is a valuable way of developing this. These can them be used as a basis for games at home and at school.

Example: Word patterns

hear   fear   beard

heard   near   pear   ear

learn   dear   wear

Older dyslexic children need a more adult approach when learning about language. They will need to use their higher level thinking skills to explore word derivations — where words come from, where our language comes from and how words are built up. This is called 'etymology'. It is a fascinating subject and, as a bonus, children will gain new historical and geographical knowledge.

Skills for Spelling

The skills which are essential for good spelling can be summarized as follows:

- Adequate vision and hearing

- An awareness of the alphabet, of the letters of the alphabet

- An understanding of the importance of vowels and their sounds

- A thorough rhyming ability

- Adequate ability to match symbols with their sounds

- An awareness and knowledge of language especially syllables

- Clear speech

- Clear cursive writing

- A good memory for words and images

Characteristic Spelling Errors

The problem is that these skills are the very ones which tend to be areas of weakness for dyslexics. Dyslexic children tend to make **characteristic spelling errors** often linked to these weaknesses. These can be summarised as follows:

- Omitting letters: 'ther' for 'there'

- Reversals of letters or word: 'wnet' for 'went'

- Shortening of the middle of words: 'happed' for 'happened'

- Basic confusions: 'crt' for 'cart'

- Purely phonic interpretations: 'becos' for 'because'

- Logical misspelling: 'skool' for 'school'

- Words that sound the same but are spelt different : 'there' for 'their'

- Muddling of letter names and sounds: 'hap' for 'happy'

- Letters in incorrect order: 'wrer' for 'were'

Further examples of these errors are given below.

In many of these errors, the rough outline of a particular word may be the same or similar to the correct word, but the inner detail is missing or it is different with some of the letters jumbled. When children are mainly or only relying on the outline of a word as a clue to its spelling and reading, visually similar words like 'house' or 'horse' can easily be confused. On the other hand, they may forget to cross 't's', and cross 'l's', instead which will completely alter the word: for instance 'taler' could be written for 'later'. The dyslexic child may do a number of inappropriate things with words or letters: reverse them, ('b' for 'd'), mirror them ('was' for 'saw') or telescope them ('rember' for 'remember'). They might put them in the wrong place ('Wenedesday' for 'Wednesday'or simply add them to the end to fill up the space to what they remember from the shape of the word is the correct length. ('caterparill' for 'caterpillar'). Another difficulty arises when the child is unsure whether there is one word or two. Is it 'a lot' or 'alot'? Is it 'about' or 'a bout'? Some **further examples of typical spelling mistakes** taken from dyslexics' writing are given in the table.

Further examples of typical spelling errors

Child's attempt	Actual word	Kind of error
taler	later	't' crossed in the wrong place.
frm	farm	Confusion between letter sound of 'r' and its name.
oneted	wanted	Phonic errors but a phonically logical spelling.
how	who	Letters not in correct sequence.
frist	first	Sequencing again.
rember	remember	Telescoping the middle of the word.
a bout	about	Not sure if its one word or two.
ct	seat	Confusion between letter name and sound.
bumgoil	gumboil	Sequencing and naming ability.
evenchilly	eventually	Phonic error possibly linked with articulation difficulty.
km	came	Letter name and sound confusion.

Child's attempt	Actual word	Kind of error
saw	**was**	Reversal of letters.
tnu	**nut**	Sequencing: right letters but wrong order.
onty	**only**	Crossed the 'l' by mistake.
slitt	**still**	Another variation of miscrossed 'ts' and 'l's'.
relay	**really**	Usually this is mainly an articulation error.
vellvit	**velvet**	Phonic error.
earport	**airport**	Mainly an articulation error.
ortigruf	**autograph**	Phonic.
sa	**essay**	Letter names confused with their sounds.
noese	**knows**	Phonic.
lime	**time**	Those 'l's' and 't's again.
me cee	**merci**	French written language confusion.
ge mapelle	**je m'appelle**	And another one.

Understanding Why Words are Spelt the Way They Are

There is only a tiny number of people who cannot spell at all, and only a few very weak spellers. Even if children make the kind of mistakes shown in the last table, it does not mean that they are hopeless at spelling and will never improve. Look for the positive. Nearly all the misspelt words in the table have most of their letters correctly chosen but sited in the wrong place. Given the right context, the reader would be able to understand what the writer meant. Here are some examples. You will probably be able to read them correctly despite the errors:

I saw the book I oneted and so I bort it.

He was relay good looking.

Our front room curtens are made of red velvitt.

She noese the right answer.

He wrote a brilliant sa on the origins of the First World War.

Spelling errors need not detract from understanding. If children make these kinds of logical error, it means that they understand the basic rule of spelling. They know that there is a relationship between the way words sound in their heads and the way they look on the page. Often when looking at children's spelling we are so concerned with the one or two letters that they use incorrectly that we forget all the letters and parts of words that are right. If a child always misspells about 10 out of every 100 words some might label him or her a bad speller. If the same child always gets 90 out of 100 sums correct we say: '90% right. Well done. You are really good at Maths!'

It is important to remember that approximately 80% of all English words are phonically regular. The spelling of 80% of words conforms to a recognised pattern, principle or rule. Understanding why these words follow patterns, principles and rules should help develop a child's ability to spell them. Learning all these rules by heart is not a successful strategy with dyslexics. If the rules mean nothing, or if their underlying pattern has not been explained, then they will be quickly forgotten. Rules need to be understood and applied.

Methods to Help Children Improve Their Spelling Skills

There are many ways for children to improve their spelling ability. But before we consider them, remember the golden rule:

CHILDREN WILL NOT LEARN TO SPELL BY COPYING OUT
LISTS OF WORDS.

Copying is not a good way of memorising spellings and building up a useful spelling vocabulary. It is literally a paper exercise. Children who are encouraged to look at words carefully, to see the patterns in words and to develop the skills needed to commit spellings to memory are the ones who are most likely to improve.

This chapter continues with some methods which will help children's spelling progress They can be used at home or at school and are relevant for any spellings which children need to learn: whether for the dreaded weekly spelling test or for the technical words specific to some secondary subjects which need to spelt quickly and automatically if the child is to succeed on the course.

Visual inspection

This is a famous method although it has many variations across the country. We call it the 'LOOK–PICTURE–COVER–PICTURE–WRITE–CHECK' method. It follows this sequence: The child must:

- LOOK at the word, then
- PICTURE the word. By 'picture' we mean the child tries to visualise the word. They try to see the word in their 'mind's eye'
- COVER the word
- PICTURE the word again

- WRITE the word and, finally,

- CHECK the word to see if it is written correctly.

The child can be given the word needed on the top of a sheet or paper. The word is then *looked* at and studied. The child then visualises or *pictures* the word in the mind. The paper is then folded to just *cover* the word. The child should then picture the word in the mind again. Then the child *writes* the word just below the fold. The two words are then *checked*. If the child's word is wrong it should not be altered. The child should begin again.

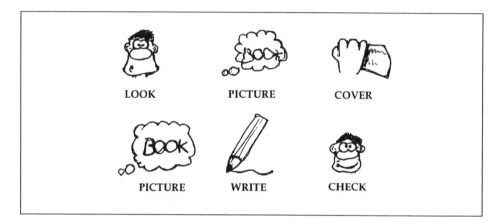

Simultaneous oral spelling (SOS)

This sounds very difficult but is actually simple to do and can be very effective. Its shortened title is SOS and it might just save the child when it comes to learning some of more troublesome irregularly spelt words. Unfortunately the downside of 80% of English words being regular is that 20% are not and these are often the most used words. (They probably became irregular because of their extensive use as the written language developed.) SOS uses a multi-sensory approach. This means that it uses all the senses it can as pathways to the memory: vision, hearing and touch. To these pathways is added the speech route. The idea is that if there is a weakness in one pathway, another can take its place. Nothing is left to chance.

Its main stages are:

HEAR IT.

SAY IT.

SEE IT.

WRITE IT.

To begin with the word needs to be written by an adult and then said. The child looks at it and also says it. The child then writes the word saying each letter as it is written down:

'please — p-l-e-a-s-e spells please'

The child then checks to see if the word has been spelt correctly. The whole process is repeated three times. It is important to make sure that the word is not copied but repeated from memory each time, so cover the word after the child has seen it and said it. The new word should then be used in a sentence. It is a useful technique to use this method for those tiresome words which your child uses frequently and always seems to get wrong. The child will probably be able to tell you what these words are. If so this will make the task more meaningful and if it is more meaningful it is likely to be successful

Simple strategies for remembering words (also known as *Neuro-linguistic Programming* (NLP))

These are very simple and effective ways of learning spellings. The child is encouraged to look carefully at a word, cover it and try to form a mental picture of it. This is the second step in the 'Look, Picture, Cover, Picture, Write, Check technique.

These strategies build on the strengths which many dyslexics have in their right brain hemisphere, strengths like colour appreciation, imagination, day-dreaming and imagery (seeing in pictures). When spelling a new word, or any tricky word, the child is prompted by asking questions which encourage looking at the word critically and in some detail. This helps to fix the mental image of the word in the child's mind.

The use of colour is recommended. A highlighting pen is ideal for this. Very few children have difficulty with all the letters in a new word to be learnt. The highlighter is used to show the child which part of the word they already know and which parts they need to concentrate on. This will allow the child — and you — to see clearly and concentrate on ways of remembering the difficult parts. This helps to reduce the load on the child's memory and increases confidence as the child is told or realises that much of each new word's spelling is already known.

The kinds of questions to ask:

(1) How many letters?

(2) Looking left to right, are there any small words in it? (for example:
there: the, here, her, he.; *knowledge*: know, no, now, owl, ledge, edge)

(3) How many vowels?

(4)   How many tall letters/small letters/descending letters are there? Tall:
       b, d, f, h, k, l, t; small: a, c, e, i, m, n, o, r, s, u, v, w, x, z; descending: g, j, p, q, y

(5)   Which parts can you spell already?

(6)   Which parts will you have problems with?

(7)   What are the letters in the word? — Say them.

(8)   Has the word got a shape? Describe it. (For instance: long and thin, short
       and tall, like a train, stumpy, skinny and so on.)

(9)   Write the word in joined writing.

(10)   Are any letters repeated (for example 'banana — b-an-an-a')?

(11)   Can you find a special way of remembering this word? (For example
       'Ne*cess*ary' has a *cess*pit in the middle!)

Mnemonics

This is a good way of remembering tricky or awkward spellings which need to be
in the memory but are difficult to keep there. It is an old favourite and is used consciously or subconsciously by most of us at some time. Mnemonics are used as pegs
on which to hang spellings. When the child needs to remember the word it is plucked
off the peg. Mnemonics are ideal for this because they use visual pictures and imagery which, in turn, use the right brain hemisphere where so many dyslexics have
strengths. The more personal, bizarre or even rude the mnemonic is the more likely it
is to get into the child's memory bank of correct spellings and stay there.

Here are some real examples collected over many years of teaching:

(1)   **Big elephants can't always use small exits** — *because.*

(2)   Sometimes a mental picture is enough to trigger a mnemonic: An
       island **is land** with sea around it.

(3)   A *piece* of **pie.**

(4)   A **U** T*u*rn!

(5)   Never bel*ie*ve a **lie.**

(6)   **You** are *you*ng.

(7)   There is a **rat** in sepa*rat*e.

(8)   **I** to the **end** will be your fr*iend*.

(9)   **O U** Lucky Duck: c*ou*ld, sh*ou*ld, w*ou*ld.

As well as using this technique to remember awkward spellings it also successful for remembering facts. For instance the colours of the rainbow be come much easier to recall with this mnemonic:

ROY Get Back In The Van:

Red, Orange, Yellow, Green, Blue, Indigo, Violet

There are many other examples of mnemonics. However, they should mean something to the child. A personal made-up mnemonic is better than one copied from somewhere else. A rude or vivid, personally made up one, is best of all.

Onset and rime

Based mainly on work by Usha Goswami (see Booklist), the Onset and Rime technique encourages children to learn reading and spelling skills simultaneuosly. By *'onset '* is meant the initial consonant sound of a word, e.g. *'s'* in *'s***op**' or *'st'* in *'s***top**' or *'str'* in *'s***trop'**. By 'rime' the vowel plus the final consonant is meant; e.g. **'op'** in these examples.

Here, the *onsets* are in italic:

b/at *c*/at *f*/at *h*/at *m*/at *p*/at *r*/at *v*/at *f*/at *s*/at

Here, the **rimes** are in bold:

br/**ing** cl/**ing** fl/**ing** r/**ing** s/**ing** spr/**ing** str/**ing** w/**ing**

The Onset and Rime technique is very simple and effective. Children are taught to read and spell a frequently used rime, such as **'old'** or **'end'**. Once this is learnt, they are shown the rime in other words: '**bold, cold, fold, gold, hold, sold** and **told**'. They very soon learn to spot the rime they have learnt, add it to the initial sound, and write or read the whole word correctly. Children find it easy to recognise the rimes they have learnt. This visual recognition reduces the load on their memory. Rimes are identical sequences of letters which occur in two or more different words. They do not always rhyme. However, there is an obvious link with rhymes, including nursery rhymes. Spot the onsets and rimes here:

Little Miss *M*/**uffet** sat on her *t*/**uffet.**

Jack *Spr*/**at** could eat no *f*/**at'**

M/**ary**, *M*/**ary**, quite *contr*/**ary**

Many reading experts emphasise the importance of singing and saying nursery rhymes to young children. The typical early-years classroom is full of songs and poetry, and storybooks which emphasise rhyme. These experiences are not just for fun and entertainment. They are vital elements of the literacy programme.

However, many dyslexic children do not pick up this kind of information as readily as other children. They need to be explicitly taught rimes and shown how they link together with onsets, to make the whole word sound. Parents and teachers can help them make this link, by using direct teaching, activities and games, like these:

(1)   Earn points by adding rimes to onsets to make as many words as possible.

(2)   Spot and say (underline or highlight), the rimes in a story, poem or song.

(3)   Read nursery rhymes and poems to them, emphasising the rhymes.

(4)   They read or recite a nursery rhyme or poem to you, with exagerated emphasis on the rimes. Or they do the same with the words of a popular record.

(5)   Cut words up into their onsets/rimes and make other words with these combinations.

(6)   Highlight rimes in words in newspapers and magazines.

With regular use of these methods, children's spelling will improve. As children's confidence grows and they start to think of themselves as good spellers, their accuracy rate will improve. It is unrealistic, though, to expect severely dyslexic children to ever become trouble-free spellers. It is far more realistic to expect them to be able to spell in a logical way even if it is not the correct spelling. In other words, *'thay mite not spell it rite but you wil kno wot they ment to say!'* Consistent accuracy is a bonus.

The Use of Information Technology in Improving Spelling

Advances in the use of information technology are rapid and widespread. These advances are of major significance to dyslexic children. We may be approaching an era when writing by hand will not be nearly as important as being able to operate a computer successfully. For instance, nearly all people who routinely use a lap-top computer for word-processing, automatically use its integral spell-checker.

The use of hand-held spell-checkers is also helping to increase spelling accuracy. Grammar checks, spell-checks, dictaphones, lap-tops, videos, audio cassettes and voice recognition programmes — all have a part to play in this new world where the dyslexic child will be freer to show his/her higher level thinking skills and maximise his/her learning potential.

Hand-held spell-checkers are now commonplace and easily available. They are portable, no larger than a calculator. They can make a real difference, especially those which are equipped with a thesaurus (a bank of words with similar meanings). They tend, though, to be rather fragile and rough games can easily damage them. They can be expensive to mend. When buying a machine check that the guarantee does cover accidental damage. We would also advise buying one with a metal case rather than a plastic are because they are much more sturdy.

New machines and software which will translate speech, spoken into a microphone, into text on a page are on the market. These will be standard in years to come. Children will then be as unlikely to use a pen to write as they now use an abacus to calculate. There may be disadvantages in this for some children, but for dyslexics, it will be a great advantage. They will be able to operate on a level playing field with their non-dyslexic peers. All children will then be able to write successfully and legibly what they have learnt. Dyslexics may even be placed in a stronger position, because when they are freed from the need to be accurate in their spelling and precise in their mental calculation, their often stronger creative and divergent thinking skills will dominate. This is not myth-making or speculation. The only factor which can stop this happening is schools themselves or the political, financial and educational systems that control schools.

Summary of Chapter 3

This chapter

- described the effects of dyslexia on children's ability to spell well;

- detailed the skills needed for spelling;

- listed spelling errors which are typical of dyslexic children;

- covered a number of methods which will improve dyslexic children's spelling skills;

- related the use of information communication technology in improving spelling.

Chapter 4

Handwriting

This chapter begins by emphasising the importance of a clear and legible handwriting style. It then describes a useful framework for assessing the strengths and weaknesses of children's handwriting with a view to designing an individual handwriting programme for them. It ends with some simple strategies for helping children overcome specific difficulties with handwriting.

Handwriting is Important

We can be judged as people by the quality of our handwriting. Some parents, teachers, pupils and prospective employers tend to see untidy or illegible handwriting as evidence of a deficiency in the writer's character and ability. At school, the content of children's written work may be undervalued because of poor handwriting. Children with an unsatisfactory script can be highly embarrassed by it, or may use it to hide an equal inability to spell. In summary, the importance of children's ability to produce an acceptable, legible script should not be underestimated.

Handwriting is a means of verbal (with words) communication between people. However, it is also a means of non-verbal (without words) communication. The quality of the script inevitably gives the reader a visual image about the hidden writer. Image is not just about what people wear, it is about the whole person. Some authorities judge that what people say counts for 7% of the impression they make, how they say it for 38% but that their appearance scores the greatest figure of 55%. If this analogy is applied to handwriting the importance of a clear and legible script becomes apparent. Rightly or wrongly the reader may make an assumption that because a piece of written work appears immature, the writer must share this immaturity. The reader will probably not take into account other reasons which might have caused the poorly presented script. These could range from difficulties with fine motor control, to tension or long-established bad habits which began with ineffective early teaching.

You may question the importance of handwriting at a time when word-processors are becoming the norm for many writers. There is computer software on the market which will type what the speaker tells it to. Why worry if children are struggling to write legibly? The machine will do it for them. Handwriting may seem to be becoming an obsolete skill.

There is an element of truth in this, and certainly the ability to write clearly at speed will not be as universally necessary in the future as it is now. However, there are many advantages of being able to write adequately which will not disappear. It gives the writer independence from machines. Technology has not, as yet, advanced far enough to cater for the unexpected need to record or communicate information. The sheer logistics of constantly carrying around a word-processor, printer and paper is not feasible. Being able to handwrite has the advantage of spontaneity — a note-pad, a scrap of paper and a pen are easily portable and come to hand in a second.

Therefore, difficulties with handwriting cannot be ignored or minimised. To do so would be to disadvantage especially those dyslexic pupils who have such problems. As with the other skill deficits covered by this book, handwriting difficulties must be positively addressed with an individual programme based on achievable targets. When beginning such a programme with children it is essential to let them know that a drastic change to their writing style is not required. One of the first things the teacher will do is to identify the good features of a child's style in order to build on them. This is to emphasise that what is needed is improvement in specific areas only. This improvement will be targeted in a series of realistic steps.

Many schools will have a policy on handwriting and presentational skills which will aim to ensure consistency of approach in all situations where children write. This will assist the child with difficulties. Many handwriting problems can be identified and resolved in an informal way by teachers working within the consistent application of a well thought out policy. There is no need to be an expert in handwriting to help children improve their writing skills. The next sections of this chapter deal with the Handwriting Action Grid or HAG. We have designed the HAG using the recommendations of Jean Alston, a handwriting specialist. (see the Booklist). This is a useful framework to help the teacher or parent identify, design and monitor specific improvement targets for each child.

The Handwriting Action Grid (HAG)

The HAG is based on a hierarchical list of skills essential for good handwriting. It has been deliberately designed to help set specific targets efficiently and effectively. For assessment purposes, it can be divided into three main sections:

(1)   The Pre-Writing Stage: The 'P' Section

(2)   The Essential Stage: The 'E' Section

(3)   The Specific Stage: The 'S' Section

The HAG sheet gives a sensible and coherent structure through which a child's handwriting style may be analysed. The intention is that when areas needing attention have been identified, targets for improvement will be set for each one. A strategy must then be devised to help children improve in these key areas so that they can reach the targets. Progress towards the targets will be entered on the action grid.

Only one target should be aimed for at any one time. Ideally this will be one whose achievement is almost guaranteed — with effort from the children — so that they may begin with success. It is important that targets are prioritised in a way which is achievable and realistic. To improve their style of handwriting requires high levels of motivation. Children must really want to improve. This will only happen if they can see they have been set targets which will stretch them but which they can reach. It is a partnership between the adult and the child, with a view to finding jointly a reason for improving, as well as an efficient and effective way of doing it. A blank Handwriting Action Grid is shown below.

THE HANDWRITING ACTION GRID (HAG)		
Name Age		Date
'P' STAGE Left/Right: 1. Position of the body 2. Paper position 3. Pen/pencil hold		**COMMENT**
'E' STAGE 4. Printing/Cursive script: 5. Writes on the line 6. Crosses 't' and dots 'i' 7. Speed of writing		
'S' STAGE 8. Slant of the letters I ///// \\\\\ 9. Size of the letters in relation to each other. 10 Space of the letters and between the words 11. Shape of the letters		
Target Signed Date		

The 'P' Section — pre-writing section

This section helps to assess children's readiness to write before pen is put to paper. It is concerned with position: the position of the body when writing (posture), the position of the hand on the pen/pencil (grip) and the position of the paper when writing, in relation to left- or right-handedness.

It is important that children are seated comfortably at a desk or table. Ideally they will be able to place both feet firmly on the ground or a foot rest. Heads should not be propped up with the spare hand. Instead the non-writing hand should be used to gently hold and balance the paper. Slouching, crouching and generally bad posture should be observed and commented upon.

The pen/pencil grip

There is no definite rule about the advisability of using either a pen or pencil. Personal preference plays an important part. Some children prefer a biro or roll-point pen, others a pencil, still others a fountain pen. Biros must be chosen carefully as some types can produce a harsh, thin line which does not help clarity. Roll-points are fashionable with children and for many produce a pleasing effect. However, we would recommend cartridge or ink pens as they give a good depth of writing. Here, again though, care must be taken over choice of nib with personal preference a major factor. Some children will only write in pencil because they consider it to be faster and neater. They should be encouraged away from this. They need to develop the ability to write with a pen, because this will probably be a requirement in the secondary school, if not the later primary school years. However, do not forcefully insist that only one type of writing instrument be used. Encourage them to try different types over a period of time and keep samples of their writing with each so that they can make an informed choice as to the best one for them. For the rest of this chapter, we will assume a pen is being used.

Keeping a correct grip on the pen is essential. In the right-hand grip the pen is held between the thumb and the index finger (the one that points), with the middle finger underneath to help it. It is recommended that the index finger is nearest to the writing nib for maximum pen control. Ideally the pen should also point towards the upper arm and shoulder. Do try and persuade your child not to hold the pen too close to the end or too tightly. They are both as bad as one another and either will produce tight and tense writing. The grip should be firm but relaxed enough to allow the hand to move with ease.

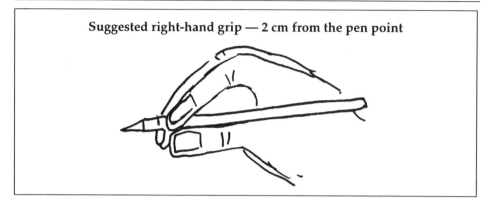

Suggested right-hand grip — 2 cm from the pen point

Left-handed children should hold the pen approximately 3 cm from its point (see diagram on the next page). They should be able to see the pen as it writes. Some left-handers occasionally write with a hooked grip. This looks very awkward and cumbersome and can cause the writing to be smudged and their hands to tire quickly. This should be gently corrected by explaining that problems can occur when writing like this. It is usually enough to stress the smudges and tired hands which result from using this grip. One way of helping them to break this habit is to use a chalkboard and easel or wall-mounted white board and pen. It is extremely difficult to write on these surfaces with a hooked grip. When they realise this, encourage them to explore other techniques. In doing so you may convince them that they are able to write with another grip and hopefully persuade them of the advantages of doing this. A good tip for the left-hander is to sit to the left of a table or double desk. In that way they have plenty of room for movement with less chance and opportunity to annoy or disturb their classmates when writing. In this position, the left and right arms and elbows of a right- and left-handed pair sitting together will not clash.

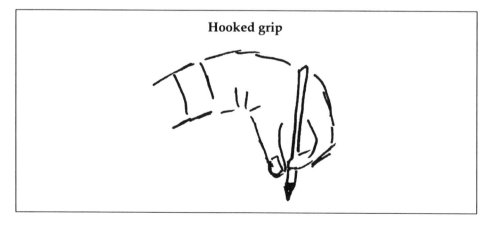

Hooked grip

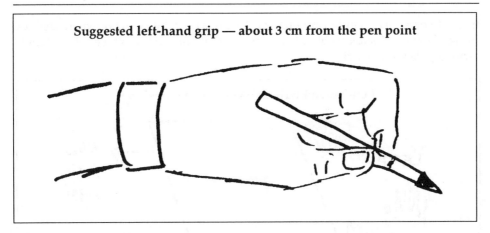

Suggested left-hand grip — about 3 cm from the pen point

The position of the paper

Having the correct position of the paper in relation to the position of the writer and the desk is vital. A right-handed pupil should have the paper slightly tilted to the left, with the left-hand acting as a gentle balance and anchor, holding the paper steady.

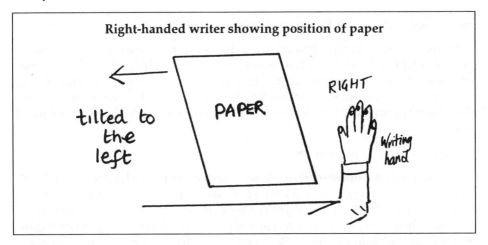

Right-handed writer showing position of paper

Conversely, the left-handed writer should have the paper slightly tilted to the right with the right hand acting as a gentle balance and anchor. Paper position is very important for left-handers because correct placement allows children to see what is being written as they write it. If they habitually use the wrong position, children should be reminded and encouraged to use the correct one. Another advantage is that it is harder to adopt the hooked grip with the paper in the right position. All teachers at school will need to reinforce attempts by children who are trying to break bad handwriting habits. This is where, by laying down guidelines for teachers in all subjects about correct position and grip, a whole school hand-writing policy is so vital.

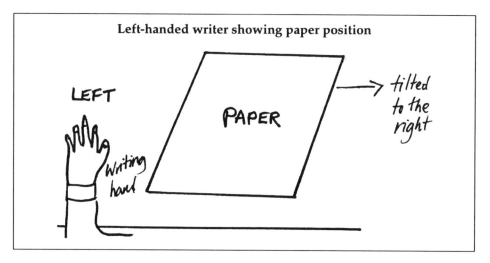

Left-handed writer showing paper position

The 'E' Section — The Essential Stage

This stage targets cursive (joined-up) writing. It is recommended that a cursive script is taught to dyslexic children as early as possible. It helps them develop that natural left to right movement across the page which is central to writing. It also encourages and gives practice in linking those letters which often occur together. This assists spelling. The following are **examples of letters which are often linked together:**

ing ed dge age tion dis re ten ion er

Cursive writing encourages children to see words as words and not simply individual letters grouped together. It helps them to see words as units with identity and meaning. It also develops a stronger sense of space. Seeing words as whole units will assist them to write with correct spacing. Some children have persistent difficulties with this skill, running letters into each other. Wrong spacing can make writing virtually illegible:

Wron gspaci ngcan mak e writ ing virtu ally ill egib le!

Cursive writing is an efficient use of movement and time. This is mainly because children do not have to take the pen off the paper and return it as often as with print-ing. In turn this reduces the number of times they have to think about the right direction for each letter or where to begin writing it. It becomes an automatic skill. **There are three main types of joined handwriting.**

(1)   The straight join, linking letters horizontally from left to right:

ooo   or   owr   owto

(2)   The diagonal join, linking letters with a diagonal stroke from left to right, bottom to top:

quest can   queen ear

(3)   The round join, linking letters from left to right with a round movement:

cad   cod   icicle

Initially, when children learn a cursive script, there is a tendency to print. This is because, at first, they feel that printing is quicker and neater than their early attempts at linking letters. This is natural, so expect a little resistance when the switch is made. With encouragement, practice, determination and, most important of all, motivation, the change can be made. This is true of secondary-age children who have developed a habit of printing. With perseverance, the habit can be overcome and an age-appropriate hand produced. This is important. A cursive script is much more useful to the child when meeting the demands of the secondary curriculum.

An example of a 11-year-old still printing

Monday 3 June
Saturday morning

Saturday morning I went to Mold at 10:30. First we went in to Woolworth to have a look round But we, did not find eny think so we went in to Boots so we buy sum things in the so then we look round the markets then I went home

From the previous example you can see that this boy's original writing looks immature and there are some badly formed letters. As he gets older, he will inevitably be required to write more and at greater speed. Without attention now, the quality of his writing will then decline further. He will also become increasingly aware that the writing of other children looks more mature and sophisticated than his own. That will be no small matter for young, self-conscious, emerging teenagers. The parent or teacher needs to persuade them not to abandon their style of writing but to improve it. They need to be assured that improvement is realistic and achievable without undue discomfort. The example below is the same boy's script, three months later. He had been working on one achievable target: to use a cursive script for all his lessons. At first resistant, the idea that his writing looked immature motivated him to change.

The same boy's handwriting three months later

Another target which can be easily identified and worked on, sometimes producing spectacular results for little effort, concerns the need to write on the line. This is readily apparent and can be easily assessed and addressed. Children who do not write on the line have often drifted into this habit. As a result, their writing looks careless and ill considered. Often all they need is their attention drawn to the habit, an assurance they can write on the line and a specific target at which to aim. Setting such targets — i.e. 'Write on the line in all lessons.' — can have an instant impact with immediate results — especially if all teachers encourage this in their lessons.

Another part of the essential stage is concerning with dotting 'i's' and crossing 't's'. Many children have difficulty remembering to do this. Once again, it only involves setting a relatively minor target, but achieving it can greatly improve legibility as these **common handwriting errors** show:

taler = later ('t' crossed in the wrong place)

lime = time ('t' not crossed)

slitt = still ('t' crossed in the wrong place)

falher = father ('t' not crossed)

Speed of writing is the final area to be considered in this section. As children get older the curriculum demands more and more writing at a greater speed. Depending on the age of the class, teachers will assume a certain minimum speed of writing. If children are significantly slower than this expected speed, the potential for problems is clear. A slow, laborious writer may be too tense or anxious or too preoccupied with perfection or fear of failure. Whatever the cause, they will either be forever catching up or will have no completed pieces of work. Equally, if in an attempt to keep up, children write too fast for their skill level, their script may become illegible. Some children write too fast because their minds work more rapidly than their hands, others simply because they want to finish before the rest and be first to complete their work.

The ability to write legibly at an adequate speed is an important skill. Children with difficulties in this area will need their individual speed assessed with an appropriate target set for improvement. This target will need to balance legibility against speed. It is important that quality is maintained but not at the expense of reasonable speed.

Slow writers can be given exercises to increase speed. Usually these are timed exercises with children working against the clock to improve on the time taken for a set amount of writing. The challenge may be twofold. Firstly, to achieve an overall time target, say how much can be written legibly in 2 minutes. Secondly, they can be told to improve on their previous performance with each subsequent attempt.

Or children might be given a choice of two sentences to write. Examples might be:

I like jam for tea.

The cat sat on the box.

These are simple sentences which do not rely on good spelling skills. Therefore, the children can concentrate on forming letters and words at speed. The emphasis is on producing correctly formed cursive script at speed. They are given 2 minutes to write the chosen sentence. At the end of this time, the number of letters and words formed correctly is counted. It is important to change the sentences regularly so that there is practice with different words and letter combinations. Each time the pupil should record the score. Self-recording against targets is a successful and highly motivating experience for most children. This is because children will not feel threatened by the rivalry of siblings or peers. Instead they have instant feedback with, hopefully, a feeling of success that the new score is an improvement on last time. Nothing succeeds like success.

Some children have the opposite problem. They write too quickly for their script to be legible. They share this difficulty with some professional people who, for a variety of reasons, write too rapidly. The consequences of this may vary. The doctor whose illegible prescription caused the wrong drugs to damage a patient may be sued for negligence. The teacher, who exhorts a child to write more neatly but records this in a hand so illegible the child cannot read it, is in contrast not providing a role model for the child to emulate.

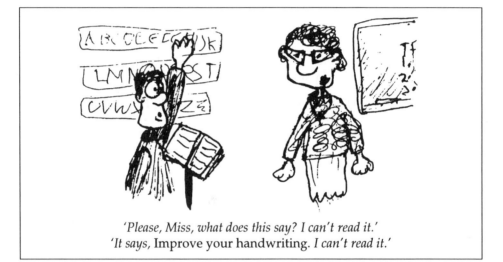

'Please, Miss, what does this say? I can't read it.'
'It says, Improve your handwriting. I can't read it.'

Speed of hand, whether too fast or too slow, can be the extra factor which causes the writing of some dyslexic children to collapse under the strain of a timed test or examination. Extra time for National Curriculum Tests can be allocated by a school to its dyslexic pupils to help them avoid this kind of pressure. Secondary schools can provide extra time for their significantly dyslexic pupils during GCSE examinations and 'A' levels (see p.164). Schools should also allow extra time for their own internal examinations. This is not a concession to the children concerned. It is a right and one which allows them to show what they know on a fairer basis with other children. Some children may be granted extra time but do not use it. However, the mere fact that they can take extra time if they need to, may reduce their stress and cause them to write at a more reasonable rate than would otherwise have happened.

The 'S' Section — The Specific Stage

This section deals with a number of handwriting skills in turn. It begins with the need to create spaces between letters and word. Then it deals with the angle at which letters should be formed. Following this the size of letters is covered, particularly those letters which rise above the line or descend beneath it. Finally the correct shaping of letters is described.

Spacing is dealt with first. This refers to the spaces between words as well as between letters. As we showed in an earlier example, uneven spacing between words can cause many problems for the reader. Here is another badly spaced sentence. It is very familiar to you, though maybe not when it is written like this:

Th ecatsa tont hem at.

This example can be shown to children to help them understand the importance of good spacing. If they realise this, they may be more likely to space correctly themselves. However, some children do not know how to do so. They need to be taught a strategy to show them how. The aim of this is to try to get children spacing automatically, without consciously having to think about it. Writing in a cursive style should resolve any problems with spacing between letters. The idea of leaving a space between words is very straightforward. When it is pointed out to them, most children grasp this quickly and easily. They simply need to be shown how wide to make each space, to be given a simple aid to their memory for doing so and then set an appropriate improvement target. One easy way is for children to use the width of their pen as a guide for the width of the space.

Rivers of space   difficulties

Some children, with very uneven and erratic spacing, create 'rivers of space' in their writing:

This phenomenon has not been fully explained. Some children have difficulties when reading the printed page and complain about seeing 'rivers' on it. One explanation is that they may be sensitive to the glare of the white page in contrast to the black of the print. As a result, they perceive the print to be moving. It jiggles about, causing these 'rivers' to appear as spaces between words.

Incorrect spacing of words can produce the same effect for the reader. However, the cause here is less likely to be glare off the page. It tends to be simply the inadequate or uneven spacing itself. This will be discussed later in Chapter 7.

Slope or slant of letters/words

A cursive script requires that words should either be upright or slope consistently to the right or left.

\\\\\\\\\\\\\\\ or //////////////

The direction does not matter. Its consistency does. All letters should be uniform in terms of direction and being parallel with each other.

Size of letters

The next consideration is the size of letters, their size in relation to each other. In this context letters are categorised as being lower case (not capitals) or upper case (capitals). They may also be ascenders (they have upright tails) or descenders (they have hanging tails).

Lower case

b c d e f g h i j k l m n o
q r s t u v w x y z

Upper case

A B C D E F G H I J K L M

Ascenders

b d f h k l t

Descenders

f g j p q y

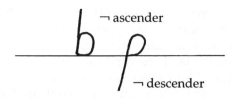

Note that 'f' ascends and descends. The difference between the 'b' and the 'p' is the ascending/descending stroke. When we read we tend to concentrate on the top half of words. Without clear ascenders this is difficult. **Lower case letters must be half way or mid zone to the ascending letters**.

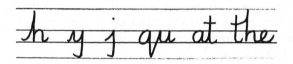

Care should also be taken with the size of capital letters. They are larger than lower case letters. Difficulties in letter size are easy to identify. Realistic targets then need to be set.

The only difference between the letter 'p' and the letter 'b' is the ascender or descender. A multi-sensory approach may help children distinguish between the two. Letters backed with sandpaper, plastic or wooden letters can be used. They allow children to feel the difference between an ascender and a descender as they see it and say the letter name or sound.

An activity to help children distinguish between letters

(1) Different sized plastic or wooden letters can be placed in a bag.

(2) Children are then asked to pull out an upper or lower case letter, or one with an ascender and so on.

(3) Letters can be pulled randomly.

(4) Children class them appropriately as they come.

(5) Related activities would be to match upper and lower case letters and grouping letters by size or descender/ascender.

Many children are taught to write using ruled paper. The width between lines is referred to as the *feint*. Initially they will use a wide feint. As control over size is attained and fine motor control develops, narrower feint will be introduced. If there are severe problems in this area then the use of tactile paper may help. The top and bottom lines are raised so children can feel them. This form of multi-sensory working will help children feel where the tall letters and the limits of the small letters. There are no hard and fast rules. Children vary. Some will need guidelines for ascenders and descenders for a long time. Others may not need them at all.

Getting the size right can make a significant difference to the legibility and clarity of writing. This is another target which can produce rapid and dramatic results. As with all these targets, however, it is important that the new skills which children learn are transferred to other situations. It is of no use if they produce a perfect hand with one teacher or their parents but then revert to their bad habits in other lessons. Their new skills need to become an automatic part of their handwriting style. This will require perseverance over time for many children. To maintain their improvements they will need to be well motivated and really wish to develop a style of writing appropriate to their age and ability.

Shape of letters

Getting the shape of letters right is the most problematic area for the non-specialist to handle because the child will need more individual attention. The main rules to follow seem rather obvious but many dyslexic children do not routinely follow them. The rules are that closed letters should be closed and open letters should be open.

Closed letters should look closed

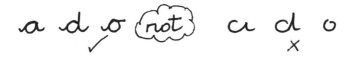

Open letters should look open

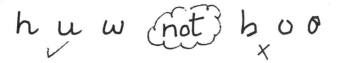

Care should also be taken with the direction of letters

b/d   p/d   m/w   u/n   s/z
→←   ↓↑   ↑↓   ↑↓   →←

Letters are grouped together according to their formation

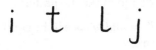

(a)   These letters all begin the same way and go in a left direction

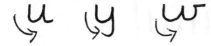

(b)   These are all curving letters.

i   t   L   j

(c)   These letters are straight and start at the top.

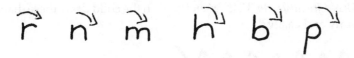

(d)   These letters are open and must look open and curve right from below.

(e)   These letters curve to the right.

k   v   x   z

(f)   These letters have straight lines with no curves.

Trouble-shooting errors with letter formation

Handwriting specialists have devised checklists and suggestions to help correct errors in the shaping of letters. The following are the most helpful:

Problem: *The child has difficulty forming the letters: 'b', 'h', 'n', 'm', 'p', and 'r'. See if the* child can produce the following pattern smoothly and easily.

mmmmm

If not, practice is needed in this push pattern handwriting movement.

Problem*: The child has difficulty with these letters: 'l', 't', 'u' and 'y'.* See if the child can reproduce the following pattern smoothly and easily.

uuuuuuuu

If not, practice the pull handwriting movement needed to make the pattern.

Problem*: The child has difficulty writing the letters 'g', 'l', 'p' and 'y'.* See if the child can produce vertical or upright patterns smoothly and easily:

If not, practice is needed.

Problem*: The child has difficulty with 'k', 'v, 'x' and 'z'.* Can the child draw these diagonal patterns smoothly and easily?

WWWWWW

If not, then practice if needed.

Problem*: The child has difficulty with the formation of these letters, 'a', 'c', 'd', 'g', 'o' and 'q'.* Can the child draw the 'c' shape smoothly and easily and do they know how to close and open the shape?

O C O C a

If not, then they need to practice this sequence:

It is best to teach the shape and formation of problem letters in a multi-sensory way. This is an effective means of thoroughly installing them in children's memory. When they have been able to simultaneously see them, hear them, touch them and speak them it is more likely that they will remember how to write them. This can be achieved in a number of ways: The following are **some multi-sensory methods for learning formation/shape**:

(1) Say it as they see it as they write it in the air with big arm movements.

(2) Say it as they see it as they draw it on their palms with small finger movements.

(3) Say it as they see it as they write in rice or sand or anything else.

(4) Say it as they see it as they feel it in a bag.

(5) Say it as they see it as they write it around a large letter projected on a wall.

(6) Say it as they feel it as they visualise it as someone writes it on their back.

An Equation for Good Handwriting

The HAG sheet is useful for the busy parent or teacher because it provides them with a framework on which to hang targets. Another way of remembering the key elements of good handwriting is to express the HAG sheet in the form of an equation (explained more fully in the figure):

$$\frac{3p+4s}{C} = \frac{it}{Sp}$$

An equation for good handwriting

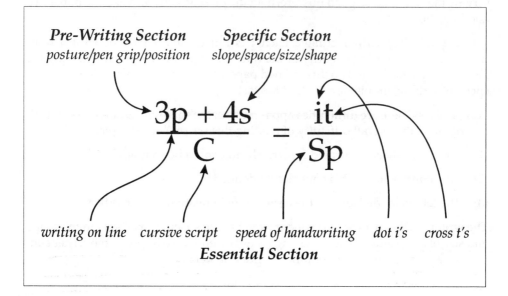

Applying the HAG Framework

Two worked examples follow:

Example A: Alan. The following script is mature and easy on the eye for skimming, but is hard to decipher in places.

Pre-Writing Skills: The HAG framework would record no difficulties here. Observing the writer had a good posture, held the pen correctly and had the paper in a good position.

Essential Skills: The script is cursive. Each 'i' is dotted and each 't' crossed. The writing is on the line for the majority of the time although there is a tendency to drift away from the horizontal on this unlined paper. There could be a problem with the speed of writing, in this case writing too fast.

Specific Skills: There are difficulties apparent with the shape of certain letters which contribute to the overall difficulty of reading this script. For example:

(1)   The 'h' in 'sheer' is formed incorrectly and could be confused with a 't'.

(2)   The letter 'w' in 'with' is not clearly defined.

(3)   The letters in 'the' are not the correct size in relation to each other.

The writer of this script would benefit from having specific targets set in the shape and size of some letters. Drastic change is not essential. To improve the writer simply needs to concentrate on refining his present style.

THE HANDWRITING ACTION GRID (HAG)		
Name *Alan*	Age	Date
'P' STAGE		**COMMENT**
Left/Right:	Right	
1. Position of the body	Fine	
2. Paper position	Fine	
3. Pen/pencil hold	Fine	
'E' STAGE		
4. Printing/Cursive script:	Fine	
5. Writes on the line	Mostly	Tends to drift on unlined paper? Monitor.
6. Crosses 't' and dots 'i'	Fine	
7. Speed of writing	?	Monitor writing at speed.
'S' STAGE		
8. Slant of the letters I ///// \\\\\	Fine	
9. Size of the letters in relation to each other.	No	Some problems here. Target needed.
10 Space of the letters and between the words		Fine
11. Shape of the letters		Target needed for 'h' and 'w'.
Target Priority One: Size of letters; Priority Two: correct formation of 'h' and 'w'.		
Signed	Date	

Example B: Jim.   This has been written by a bright, teenage dyslexic boy.

Pre-Writing Skills: He is right-handed and sits to write in a relaxed manner with a good posture. The paper is correctly positioned when writing. He appears to hold his pen too tightly at times although his actual grip is fine. The tension of his grip needs to be monitored and, if it persists, be targeted.

Essential Skills: The writing is cursive and mostly on the line. The script is mature. There is a possibility that it could deteriorate when the writer is put under pressure to write at speed. This needs to be monitored.

Specific Skills: There is some inconsistency with the sloping of letters. The word 'may' has a 'y' which slopes to the right whereas the 't' in 'then' and the 'ar' in the first word, slope slightly to the left. These should be targeted. Overall the script has a strong upright bias whose consistent use should be encouraged. The size of letters and spacing between words are problem areas. This is where the main targets should be set and addressed. Ascenders and descenders are good, but lower case letters are uneven. Words are not spaced evenly. For instance, the words on 'Often from January' are spaced too widely compared to the majority of other word spacings.

THE HANDWRITING ACTION GRID (HAG)

Name *Jim*	Age	Date
'P' STAGE		**COMMENT**
Left/Right:	Right	
1. Position of the body	Fine	
2. Paper position	Fine	
3. Pen/pencil hold	?	Tension in his grip needs monitoring
'E' STAGE		
4. Printing/Cursive script:	Fine	
5. Writes on the line	Fine	
6. Crosses 't' and dots 'i'	Fine	
7. Speed of writing	?	His writing may deteriorate when writing at speed. Monitor

'S' STAGE		
8. Slant of the letters I / / / / / \ \ \ \ \	No	Some inconsistencies; target needed here
9. Size of the letters in relation to each other.	No	Problems here; target needed
10 Space of the letters and between the words		Fine
11. Shape of the letters		Problems here, target needed

Target   Priority One: Spacing between words; Priority Two: Size of letters; Priority Three: Sloping of some letters.

Signed   Date

Some Common Handwriting Mistakes Made by Dyslexic Children

Mistake	*Example*
Starting letters in the wrong place	
Forming letters by going in the wrong direction	
Putting extra strokes on letters	
Leaving strokes out of letters	
Letters too large	
Letters too small	
Body height of letters uneven in relation to each other	
Spaces between words too small	
Spaces too large	
Spaces uneven	
Slope of letters inconsistent	
Letters do not stay on the line	
Tall letters the wrong height	
Descending letters the wrong depth	

There is no magic formula or strategy for helping children to improve each of these specific difficulties. The following process should be followed:

(1)   Explain the nature of the error.

(2)   Demonstrate how it should be done.

(3)   The child practices.

(4)   Check and repeat until correct result achieved.

(5)   Praise.

(6)   Check to ensure child is not making the error in normal writing. If so return to (1).

What are the Qualities of Good Handwriting?

Good handwriting will normally contain the following features:

- The height of the letters is consistent.

- Letters are the correct size in relation to each other.

- Closed letters are closed, e.g. 'a, d, b'

- Open letters are open, e.g. 'u, v, and y'

- Curved letters are curved and round.

- Straight letters are straight and upright.

- Spacing between letters is even and appropriate.

- Each letter is linked to the next with the correct joining stroke.

- Each 't' is crossed and 'i' is dotted.

- Ascenders are high enough to be seen.

- Descenders are low enough to be seen.

- Capital letters are sized and shaped correctly.

- The writing has been completed at a reasonable speed.

Some Final Thoughts

Handwriting is as personal to individuals as their fingerprints. It relates to a person's identity. Care must be taken not to criticise it in an overtly negative way. This is one reason for stressing that it is improvement we seek, not major changes to style.

Some dyslexic pupils with severe handwriting difficulties may be called *'dysgraphic'*. This means that they have a specific difficulty with handwriting. The severely dysgraphic child may have difficulties in many or all of the areas described in this chapter. Some of these children may eventually need to turn to alternative ways of recording their work in school. A word processor is an obvious option here. Pupils who genuinely need these machines because they cannot improve their handwriting to a level adequate for school are in a small minority. They are the exception to that majority of dyslexic pupils who can and do improve their handwriting to an adequate proficiency through the use of appropriate, well planned and implemented targets.

Mind Map of Handwriting Legibility

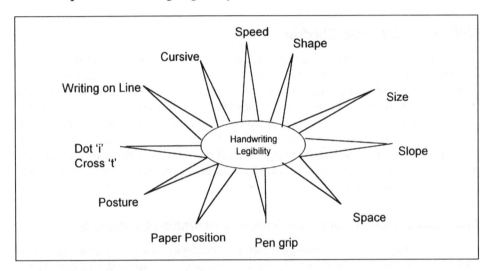

Summary of Chapter 4

This chapter

- showed how important handwriting is for children's progress;

- introduced a new way of analysing children's handwriting — the Handwriting Action Grid or HAG;

- showed how children can be encouraged to develop a clear, effective cursive style of handwriting;

- looked at common handwriting errors made by dyslexics.

Chapter 5
Writing

This chapter deals with an area which most dyslexic children find very difficult: getting their thoughts and feelings down on paper. It answers such questions as: How can they be helped to overcome these difficulties with writing? What written tasks are most difficult for them? Which parts of the writing process need to be targeted for them by school and home?

Writing and Dyslexic Children

Most dyslexic children find writing a daunting task. It is as though, for dyslexics, the word 'writing' should have an attached government health warning. Pupils who are otherwise articulate and able, who can speak their thoughts fluently and coherently, easily lose their way when faced with a blank page and asked to fill it with those same thoughts. The gap between what they know and how they show what they know to others is at its widest when dyslexic children write. This does not mean the physical act of handwriting. What it does mean is the ability to convey thoughts and feeling in extended writing at a level appropriate to children's ability, experience and knowledge.

Teaching Children about the Structure of Written Language

Written language can be broken down into component parts or chunks. A key strategy for dyslexic writers is to learn how language is chunked and how these chunks may be used to build up their own writing. A useful analogy is to think of how we approach eating a bar of chocolate. These bars tend to be pre-formed into chunks. If you try to eat the entire bar at one go, it will prove awkward and indigestible. It could hurt your mouth because the bar in its entirety will be too big to handle at one go. However, if it is broken along the pre-formed lines into bite-sized chunks, the bar can be eaten with ease. Also the eater will enjoy it and return for more. A successful and pleasant experience is more likely to be repeated than an unsuccessful and unpleasant one.

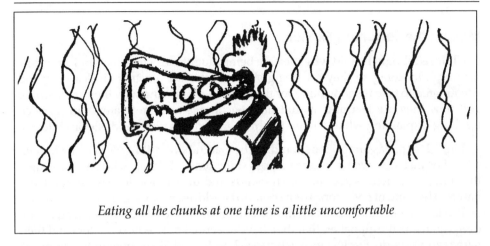

Eating all the chunks at one time is a little uncomfortable

Teaching dyslexic children to write follows a similar strategy. The structure of written English is broken down into its component parts. Children are then explicitly taught the relationships between these parts, how they fit together and work together. Finally they are shown how to use this knowledge in their own writing. The following figure demonstrates this.

The building blocks of writing

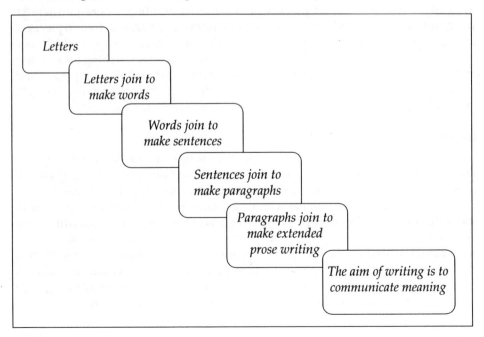

Letters

Letters join to make words

Words join to make sentences

Sentences join to make paragraphs

Paragraphs join to make extended prose writing

The aim of writing is to communicate meaning

Making the Teaching Explicit

Children should be told why they are being taught particular facts or in a particular way. In doing so they are being shown respect as partners in learning and encouraged to take responsibility for that learning. Knowing why they are learning and how they are learning should help encourage and motivate them. Explicit teaching, explaining what you are teaching and why is vital for dyslexic children.

Linked to this, assumptions should not be made about children's existing knowledge. For instance, we have come across some older children who have assumed that lower case letters say the letter sounds and upper case letters say the letter names. This kind of basic confusion needs to be addressed and resolved. It is an easy task to target, once it has been identified as a problem. Do not assume, because children can recite the alphabet, that they have a secure knowledge of letters and their names and sounds. For instance, letters such as 'g' and 'j' are frequently confused. Alternatively, the letters at the end of the alphabet may be relatively unfamiliar because of infrequent use. Often children may not be able to associate the name of every letter with its corresponding sound. This kind of knowledge should be checked thoroughly at the beginning of any teaching programme. The foundation needs to be sound so that it can be built upon safely.

The rationale for teaching dyslexic children to write fluently is to take them through a carefully stepped process, moving from building letters into words, words into sentences, and sentences into paragraphs, and paragraphs into pieces of extended prose. Children are given a straightforward structure upon which they can 'hang' their own writing. Their ability to write, to have something informative and interesting to say, is taken for granted. What they are taught is a simple support system to structure that writing, a framework which will help them write at length in a coherent and logical style. This framework will now be explained.

Letters

Our writing system is based on an alphabetic script. The letters of this script are the basic building blocks of the writing process. Close familiarity with, and knowledge of, these letters is essential. Children should be encouraged to have an interest in letters. They need to be familiar with their form, sound and feel; their position in the alphabet, their relationship to other letters and the frequency with which they are used together. It is very important that young children are aware that letters have names as well as sounds and that these are firmly grasped along with their visual image. If this knowledge is secured in the memory with a visual peg such as a clue word or picture, then it is more likely to transfer into children's long-term memory and become part of their personal store of words or lexicon.

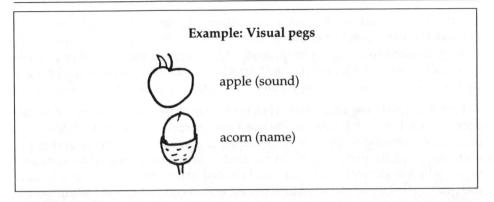

Example: Visual pegs

apple (sound)

acorn (name)

Encouraging children to associate an image of the letter with its sound or name will give them a visual peg to hang their knowledge on. This will help them remember and recall it.

It is also important for children to acquire a knowledge of the structure of the alphabet. This will increase the efficiency of their writing by improving time management. For instance, it will improve their ability to use a dictionary speedily. To do this they must know within which part of the dictionary particular words are likely to be found. Knowledge of the four quartiles of the dictionary helps here. Dictionaries can be mentally divided into four roughly equal sections, known as quartiles: A–D, E–L, M–R and S–Z. A working knowledge of the four quarters in which particular initial letters will be found means that children can quickly eliminate the other three quartiles or 75% of the possible words in the book. A useful mnemonic to help children remember these quartiles is this:

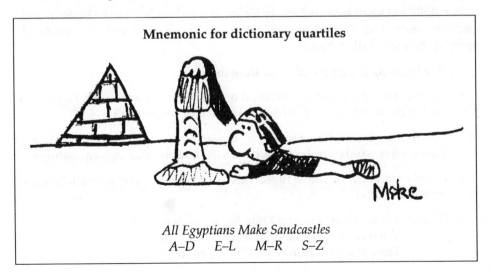

Mnemonic for dictionary quartiles

All Egyptians Make Sandcastles
A–D   E–L   M–R   S–Z

If they have this information in their automatic memory, children can, with practice, quickly find the section of the dictionary in which it is located. This is a useful strategy towards speeding up the process. Many teachers, parents and pupils are only too aware of the alternative: the frustration of the child having to go through the entire alphabet in either a song or chant to locate the position of a certain letter.

Learning how to use a dictionary is an exercise in narrowing down the available options until there is only one left: the word you are seeking. Words are placed in a dictionary according to the alphabetic sequence of their letters. When seeking a particular word, the first thing children must do is to find the section which contains words which begin with the target word's initial letter. Once this is located, they then have to find the actual word by referring to its second letter and finding words which share that letter. When these words are found the third letter is used until, by a process of elimination the actual word is found. (We know we are teaching grandmothers egg sucking here but our intention is to show how it should be explained to children.) In terms of children's learning, **a clear sequence for learning how to find a word in a dictionary** is followed in teaching this process:

(1)   Learn the sequence of the letters of the alphabet.

(2)   Learn the range and sequence of letters in each quartile.

(3)   Learn how to find the section for each letter by using the first and last words on each page.

(4)   Learn how to use the second letter to narrow it down.

(5)   Learn how to use the third letter to narrow it down and so on.

The skills and knowledge necessary for rapid word finding can be built up with games including timed activities against the clock some sample **activities for developing dictionary skills** follow:

- Word-finding games based on beating the clock.

- Linking 'find me' questions to board or computer games; i.e. the reward for finding the word means you can shake the dice or go up a level.

- Classifying games which test knowledge as well as word finding skills; e.g. 'Find me five words which are 'animals — feelings — geographical features'.

- Timed questions: 'You have 10 seconds to find me the quartile which contains the word "rabbit".'

- Quizzes: On what page would I find the word 'wizard'?
    What does 'incredible' mean?
    How many meanings does the word 'really' have?

Young children especially will enjoy these games and learn as they enjoy them. They may still have a part to play at the secondary stage. The ability to manipulate and have control over letters which games help develop is effective in building up associations between letter shape, symbol and sound.

Parts of Speech

Running parallel with this basic awareness of letters and letter patterns is the need to have a thorough knowledge of the parts of speech. Depending on their position in a sentence, words can be classified or grouped into the following parts of speech:

Part of speech	Function	Example
Common noun	A name or label for a person, place or thing	The **rabbit** lived in an ancient **warren**.
Proper noun	The specific name given to a noun	**Alan Williams** ran **Thrifty Taxis.**
Verb	A doing word, what the noun does or its action	Shalah **ran** for the gold medal.
Adverb	Adds to the meaning of the verb	She ran **quickly.**
Adjective	Describing word	The **beautiful** flowers had died.
Pronoun	Stands instead of a noun	**She** lived in an ancient warren. **He** ran Thrifty Taxis.
Conjunction	Joining words which link parts of a sentence	He lived in the town **and** died in the town.
Preposition	Tells you where things are in relation to others	She went **in** the room. He was Prince **of** Wales.

An understanding of the function of these parts of speech and how words change according to that function is invaluable in building up writing skills. With knowledge the child can develop a broad base upon which to build and manipulate words to create depth and colour in their writing. The mind map on p.106 illustrates the range and purpose of the key parts of speech which the child needs to learn. The revised English National Curriculum emphasises the need to teach these concepts. This should be of assistance to dyslexic children.

Mind map for parts of speech

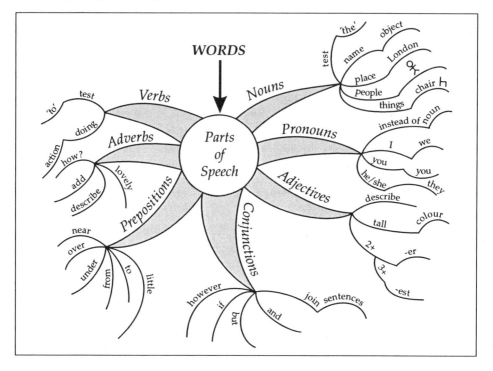

Vowels and consonants

Letters combine to make words. These words convey meaning and need to be correctly spelled. Dyslexic children need to be shown how letters and groups of letters actually combine to make words. Fundamental to an understanding of the building process is the knowledge that the letters can be classified into the two distinct groups of vowels and consonants. This needs to be accompanied with a knowledge of the importance and function of each distinct group. In case you are not sure, these are the two groups:

Vowels = a e i o u (y)

Consonants = b c d f g h j k m n p q r s t v w x (y) z

(The general rule is that y is a consonant at the beginning of words and a vowel elsewhere e.g. In *'yacht'* the *'y'* is a consonant but in *'happy'* it acts as a vowel.)

This ability to classify letters as consonants and vowels becomes very important when working on syllables and their structure. The patterns formed by consonants and vowels help break up words into recognisable syllables. This, in turn, helps decoding skills when reading and encoding skills when spelling.

Classifying letters as consonants and vowels

cat = consonant / vowel / consonant = CVC word

dog = consonant / vowel/ consonant = CVC word

hate = consonant / vowel/ consonant / silent e = CVCE

attic = vowel/ consonant/ consonant/ vowel = VCCV

When looking for a pattern of consonant and vowels in a word, children should be taught to always begin with the first vowel in a word and mark above it. They should mark 'v' for vowel and 'c' for consonant . They should then move from this to the next vowel or vowel sound.

letter = **vccv**

pupil = **vcv**

ran = **vc**

bacon = **vcv**

eggs = **vcc**

Word structure

The structure of many words often follows a familiar pattern. As the diagram illustrates, they can have a beginning section (prefix), a middle section (root) and a final section (suffix). This is not always the case. All words have roots but some words have just a prefix and root, others a root and suffix, others just the root.

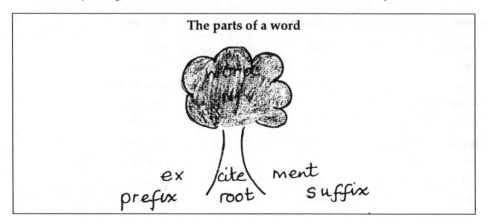

The parts of a word

ex   cite   ment

prefix   root   suffix

It is of considerable benefit for dyslexic children to be taught this structure. A knowledge and understanding of it will assist good spelling, reading and writing. An interest in word derivations fosters an interest in words themselves. An ability to analyse the make-up of a word also helps spelling skills to develop. This tuition will help develop children's understanding of the meaning of words. Each part of a word, they learn, has its own meaning. Combining these parts together will affect or qualify these meanings, often, as you will see, quite significantly. The core of a word is its root. It supports the whole structure. Many roots come from Latin or Greek. Children can become fascinated in this study of the origins of their language which will show them that the apparent idiosyncrasies of some English spellings are quite logical if you know their source. Two examples follow which show how the same root has led to whole families of words with related meanings:

Examples of word roots and their origins.

The root **'port'** comes from the Latin meaning to carry, hence words such as:

porter   reporter   export   deport   import   airport

The root **'graph'** is Greek and means write, hence words such as:

autograph   telegraph   graphology

In the table below we have listed a number of the more common Greek and Roman roots. Games in which children can combine roots with random prefixes and suffixes to form new words can be fun and instructive. Write the parts individually on small cards and then play with joining them together in different combinations. A dictionary will be needed to check some combinations, at the same time reinforcing the dictionary skills taught earlier.

Some common Latin roots of words

Root	Meaning	Example
act	do	actor
aud	hear	audience
agri	field	agriculture
amo/ami	love	amorous
annu	year	annually
aqua	water	aquarium
cap	head	captain
ceed	go	proceed
dent	tooth	dentist

Root	Meaning	Example
dict	speak	dictation
fac	make/do	factory
flex	bend	flexible
grat	please	gratitude
ject	throw	reject
jud/jus	law	justice
liber	free	liberty
loc	place	location
lum	light	luminance
mand	order	mandate
mar	sea	marine
mem	mindful	remember
min	small	miniature
mob	move	mobile
mort	death	mortality
multi	many	multitude
nat	born	native
nov	new	novice
opt	best	optimum
ped	foot	pedestrian
pel	drive	impel
pend	hang	pendant
port	carry	porter
rect	straight	erect
rupt	break	interrupt
sect	cut	intersect

Some common Greek roots of words

Root	Meaning	Example
aero	air	aeroplane
arch	chief	archbishop
ast	star	astronomy

Root	*Meaning*	*Example*
bio	life	biology
crat	rule	autocrat
chron	time	chronology
cycl	circle	cycle
demo	people	demonstration
gen	race	genocide
geo	earth	geography
gon	angle	polygon
gram	written	telegram
graph	write	autograph
hydr	water	dehydrate
log	word	dialogue
mech	machine	mechanical
meter	measuring device	thermometer
nym	name	pseudonym
opt	eye	optician
path	feeling	empathy
phobia	fear	claustrophobia
phon	sound	phonology
photo	light	photograph
poli	city	metropolitan
phys	nature	physical
psych	mind	psychology
scop	see	periscope
soph	wise	sophisticate
therm	heat	thermometer

The prefix comes before the root. Its main function is to qualify the meaning of the root. Take the word *'necessary'*. If we put the prefix *'un'* in front of this word, it reverses the word's meaning. In the same way *'behaviour'* can so easily become *'misbehaviour'* when you add the negative prefix *'mis'*. Prefixes are small but powerful as this real story shows. The following was once written by a Special Needs Adviser to all a county's headteachers:

I am confident that all schools in this county provide a wholly unsuitable education for their pupils with special educational needs.

His secretary had inadvertently added the rather insignificant prefix *'un'*. It may have been a small error but the headteachers concerned took some persuading that it was one. Some examples of prefixes are given in the table below.

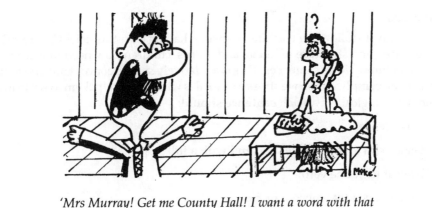

'Mrs Murray! Get me County Hall! I want a word with that Special Needs chap.'

Some common prefixes with their meanings

Prefix	Meaning	Example
bi	two	bicycle
circum	round	circumference
re	back	return
mis	wrong	mistake
pre	before	predict
sub	under	submarine
post	after	postscript
trans	across	transport
ex	out of	exit
de	down	descend
fore	before	foretell
contra	against	contradict
un	not	unhappy
in	not	incapable

In contrast to the prefix, the suffix comes after the root. Once again its main function is to qualify the meaning of the root. Two main forms of suffix are the **consonant suffix** and the **vowel suffix**.

Consonant suffixes: -ness, -ly, -ful, -ment, -tion

Vowel suffixes: -er, -ed, -ing, -able, -en, -al, -ible, -ette, -ess.

Sentences

Continuing to follow our teaching sequence, having learnt sufficient information on the nature and structure of letters and words, children now need to learn how words combine to form sentences. This is a relatively simple concept but one that is easy to over-complicate. So we stress a few rules which will help them to write in an ordered and logical way. **Each sentence should**:

(1)   make sense;

(2)   begin with a capital letter and end with a full stop;

(3)   have at least one verb;

(4)   contain one idea, concept or fact.

There is no point working on complex sentence structures and the development of complex sentences, until the child has grasped the basic concept of how a simple sentence is constructed. One useful technique is to encourage the child to draw what they think a sentence looks like. This gives you, as teacher or parent, an understanding of the child's imagery of sentence structure. Some ideas of what we mean are shown in the following figure:

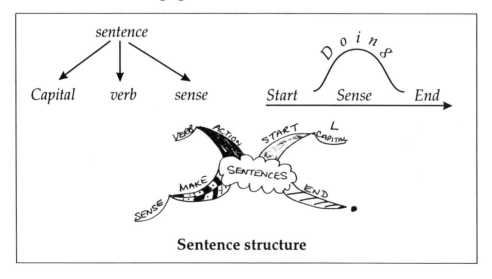

Sentence structure

We have found the following activities and exercises will help children develop the skill to write in complete sentences:

Activities which will help develop skill in sentence writing

Skill needed	Activity to help develop the skill
To limit the sentence to contain one new idea or concept or fact	(1) *Highlight the ideas in a sentence in different colours. Use newspapers and magazines.* (2) *Do the same with their own writing.*
To begin with a capital letter and end with a full stop	(1) *Highlight full stops in magazines and newspapers. See if they obey the rule with a capital letter following. Talk about why the full stop was put where it was.* (2) *Draw a mind map of the rule; e.g. see page 112.* (3) *Check their own writing to see if they follow the rule.*
To ensure that each sentence makes complete sense	(1) *Read sentences aloud carefully and discuss sense.* (2) *If more than one child is involved then they can work in pairs to proofread each other's work.*

The notion of building-up skills and knowledge via a series of carefully graded steps in learning is consistent with the principles that the British Dyslexia Association recommend for dyslexic children's programmes i.e. programmes should be thorough, multi-sensory, cumulative, structured, sequential and flexible. Given that they do conform to these principles, this section (and the ones which follow) may still seem unnecessarily restrictive and formulaic. This is especially the case when dealing with something so individual and creative as a child's ability to express him/herself on paper. The reader may be forgiven for thinking that if Shakespeare had followed these guidelines, Hamlet would have ended up looking like a 'Neighbours' script. You might object that good quality everyday writing, such as that found in many newspaper articles or children's stories, does not conform to the kind of simplicity or rigidity we appear to be recommending. We are not advocating that children should be taught to write like robots. What we are saying is that writing an extended piece of prose is a very difficult skill for most dyslexic children. They have as much to say as any other children but they need to be nurtured and supported if they are to develop the skills and self-confidence necessary to say it. One effective way of acquiring this ability and confidence is to follow a series of small, structured cumulative steps of learning. Therefore, we recommend that initially you teach children a limited set of skills and knowledge which you know they can master and which will allow them to confidently express their thoughts and ideas. It is intended that, having mastered these skills, they will progress to a more advanced and sophisticated style of writing. They are more likely to reach this level of attainment when they have had this sound, if restricted, basis upon which to build.

Paragraphs

Once sentences have been mastered, children need to be shown how they combine to form paragraphs. This is another area which can confuse dyslexic children. The problems here are similar to the ones with sentences. They may lack an awareness of the essential nature of a paragraph and may be at a loss to answer the following kinds of question:

- What is a paragraph?

- How do I start one?

- When should it end?

- How do I end it?

What is a paragraph and how do I start one?

This is best explained through imagery and example. First, tackle it visually. As in the figure, the shape of a paragraph can be drawn, illustrating how it should be indented.

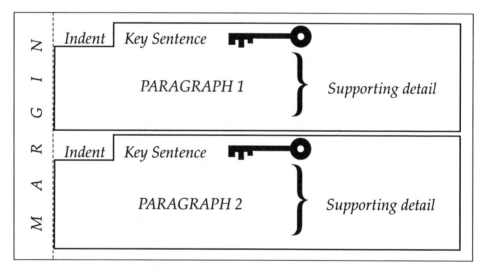

This kind of pictorial representation has been found useful by pupils taught by one of the authors. These children report that they find it easier to understand and retain the shape of a paragraph in their memory in this visual form. Their paragraphing improved once they had grasped the concepts involved.

The actual content of a paragraph also needs explicit explanation and demonstration. The usual convention is that a paragraph starts with a key sentence which defines its theme followed by other sentences which elaborate that theme with supporting explanation, detail and information. Once again, example is probably the best way to promote understanding. To do this, why not turn to the masters of prose. Take this passage from *A Christmas Carol* by Charles Dickens:

> External heat and cold had little influence on Scrooge. No warmth could warm, no wintry weather chill him. No wind that blew was bitterer than he, no falling snow was more intent on its purpose, no pelting rain less open to entreaty. Foul weather didn't know where to have him. The heaviest rain, and snow, and hail, and sleet could boast of the advantage of him in only one respect. They often came down handsomely and Scrooge never did.

This paragraph conforms precisely to our rules for good paragraphs. It begins with a key sentence which gives the reader important new information about Scrooge; namely that he was impervious to the weather. It then gives us more information and detail about this fact which illuminates and explains it. This is exactly the concept we wish to get over. You could use any source of good writing to illustrate the point, including examples within a field which you know will interest the child. Make sure the example is a good one. Unfortunately, the fact that something is in print does not mean that its paragraphing will be correct. When you have selected your paragraphs, ask children to find the key sentence and then extrapolate the main idea that the paragraph is to develop. Next, get them to show you how the rest of the paragraph achieves this. Finally, give them some simple exercises of their own to follow.

When should a paragraph end?

The answer is: when the idea posed in the key sentence has been sufficiently developed and you are ready to go on to the next idea to develop your overall aim. To illustrate this, use your sample paragraphs or discuss attempts within the child's own writing. When does Dickens finish his paragraph? The answer is when he has said all he wanted to about Scrooge's imperviousness to the elements and he now wants to move on to a new aspect of his character. Show them another paragraph to emphasise this, as here with Dickens when he continues:

> Nobody ever stopped him in the street to say, with gladsome looks, 'My dear Scrooge, how are you?'

And then he elaborates on this aspect of Scrooge's existence; his social isolation:

> No beggars implored him to bestow a trifle, no children asked him what it was o'clock, no man or woman ever once in all his life enquired the way to such and such a place, of Scrooge. Even the blind men's dogs appeared to know him; and,

when they saw him coming on, would tug their owners into doorways and up courts; and then would wag their tails as though they said, 'No eye at all is better than an evil eye, dark master!'

Again the idea stated in the initial sentence is clarified by this new detail.

The child's final query — How do I end a paragraph? — can be illustrated with both these same paragraphs. The basic principle is to end it as strongly and as pithily as possible; in a way which keeps the reader interested and emphasises the theme established by the first sentence . This is exactly what Dickens achieves with his two final flourishes:

They often came down handsomely and Scrooge never did.

No eye at all is better than an evil eye, dark master!

Extended prose writing

Finally, we come to combining paragraphs to write more extended pieces of prose. Children will need to string paragraphs together within a variety of prose forms in a logical sequence to develop a narrative or argument: essays, reports of experiments, accounts of field trips, diaries, stories, magazine articles and other assignments.

When a child's written work in a subject is not at a level appropriate to his/her ability in that subject, his/her work can be undervalued by teachers. Put another way, if they have thoroughly understood the content of a lesson, but fail to show that understanding when they put it on paper, then the teacher may assume they did not understand it. This undervaluing of dyslexic children's skills and knowledge because of recording difficulties is probably commonplace and may extend to parents, potential employers, university admission tutors and, perhaps most crucially of all, dyslexic children themselves. Children must therefore be taught techniques which will help them record and present their often high-level thinking and reasoning skills legibly. These techniques may be rather unorthodox in the classroom. Teachers must therefore be willing to accept **alternative ways of recording knowledge and understanding** to the normal form of extended prose writing. We are thinking here of the following:

- Word-processors;

- Voice recognition computer programmes (child speaks, computer writes);

- Dictaphones;

- Videotape;

- Recording in the form of notes;

- Mind maps;

- Tables/diagrams;

- Amanuensis (child speaks, someone else writes).

It can take time for teachers and parents to accept these alternative forms of recording as legitimate. It requires an understanding of their strengths and weaknesses by the pupils themselves, their parents, their teachers and the school as a whole. Schools who have formulated whole school policies for children with special educational needs including dyslexia are more likely to be able to accept and develop this kind of enlightened approach. We would not wish to over-stress this though. Modern readers and television viewers are becoming very familiar with information being presented in an extensive range of styles. Gaining information by reading extended pieces of prose writing is probably one of the least popular methods. Television, radio, CD-ROM, audio and video tape are in widespread use. In this book we have constantly sought to break up the text with tables and cartoons. We have done so in an attempt to make the information we wish to impart more accessible to you and to give variety and life to the text. From this perspective, encouraging dyslexic children to present their knowledge within a variety of formats is merely expecting them to conform to accepted norms of presentation in society itself. Maybe, rather than dyslexic children alone being encouraged to do so, it should become a routine activity for all children.

In this context, it is often difficult for dyslexic children to come to terms with writing a page on demand. It is much easier for them to have this task described in terms of it being a task which requires two or three paragraphs, each containing several sentences. This will make the task seem far less daunting. This idea of breaking down the task into 'bite-sized' chunks takes us back to the chocolate bar analogy with which we began this chapter.

Mind mapping will help children use this chunking technique more effectively. An example of a mind map devised by a dyslexic child as part of her GCSE coursework is shown in the next figure. The complete essay follows.

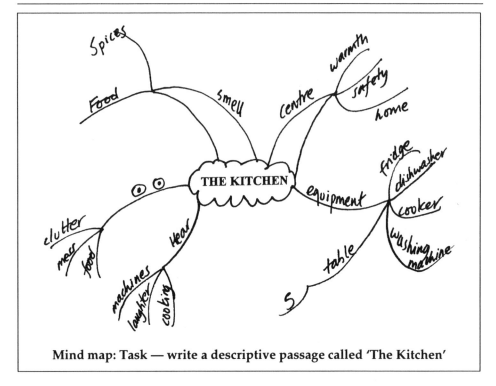

Mind map: Task — write a descriptive passage called 'The Kitchen'

The kitchen

The inviting smell of the kitchen beckoned me to enter and once again I marvelled at the chaos and disorder that mother created in this centre of our home.

In one corner of the kitchen were cramped towels, rolls of lace, assorted pens and rubbers, stacks of books, broken, chipped cups, pudding cloths and old saucepans all higgledy-piggledy stacked on the worksurfaces. The worksurfaces were strange but quaint and mother said they were her filing cabinet.

Next to the worksurfaces was my mother's larder. This too was overflowing with crockery and all kinds of exotic herbs and spices, filling the air with a peculiar smell, a mix between herbs and cereals. All different jars — fat, small, large some with lids on, others without, many cereals showing their expired by dates still lined the shelves like soldiers at attention not wanting to be thrown away. The only thing that gave them away was the boxes which had mouse nibbled holes in them.

The ancient old cooker hummed as it worked and took three hours to heat up. But it suited my mother down to the ground as it usually took her about three hours to prepare the food for the meal let alone cook it. The cooker was next to the larder with a small worksurface in between it. That worksurface was always littered with empty tins, cellophane wrappers and vegetable peelings. My mother loved this place.

The table was round and in the centre of the room with five chairs wrapped around it. My mother said it was useful as she put the peas on one side and we turned the table and the peas went to each of us in turn. This appealed to her sense of humour. The washing machine was always on the go. This was a common sound in our kitchen — the whirring we never noticed, but visitors who came always moaned about the frightful noise! My mother used to just laugh and kick it, the noise would cease instantly.

The fridge was next to the cooker on the left and the washing machine was on the right. The fridge stood tall and was seldom full. Usually there was half a pork pie that no-one wanted, two pints of milk and mouldy cheese which even a mouse rejected. My mother liked to keep things, believing that we would use it tomorrow, so she never threw anything away.

Summary of Chapter 5

This chapter

- described how written language is structured into letters, words, sentences and paragraphs;

- showed how children's writing skills can be developed by using this knowledge;

- described alternative ways in which children can record their thoughts and ideas;

- described how mindmaps can help children plan and structure their writing.

Chapter 6
Numeracy

This chapter gives a broad overview of children with specific difficulties in mathematics. It describes in general terms some typical strengths and weaknesses of the dyslexic child in the subject. We stress that several aspects of traditional mathematics methodology and mathematical language are not very compatible with the dyslexic child's learning profile. This chapter is intended mainly to raise awareness, give some basic ideas about teaching methods and indicate where further information can be found.

An Overview of Specific Difficulties with Mathematics

There is no automatic link between dyslexia and difficulties in mathematics. Some children's problems are restricted to literacy, some to numeracy and some are affected in both areas. It has been suggested that about 11% of children are excellent at mathematics but that between 40–60% may experience some type of mathematical difficulty. Children who have a significant specific difficulty with mathematics are sometimes said to be experiencing *'dyscalculia'*. Another accepted term for this is **'specific learning difficulties (dyscalculia)'**. Translated from the Greek, 'dyscalculia' simply means a difficulty with numbers. We will refer to pupils with this condition as 'dyscalculic'. This chapter will deal with two types of children who have difficulties with mathematics. In the first group are dyslexic children whose dyslexia also causes them some basic mathematical problems similar to those they experience with literacy, such as weak short-term recall or sequencing skills. In the second group are children with a significant specific learning difficulty with mathematics alone. These are the children who are dyscalculic. All of this chapter will apply to the first group. While the chapter should help with meeting the learning needs of dyscalculic children, they will almost certainly require greater depth and breadth of treatment than we cover and further reading is given at the end of the book

Fortunately, dyscalculic children usually only tend to have a specific weakness in certain aspects or areas of mathematics. It is unlikely that all their mathematical ability will be weak. Their difficulties will tend to be restricted to specific areas of mathematics skill and knowledge. In this context, mathematics can be sub-divided into several related categories: arithmetic, algebra, geometry and trigonometry. In its broadest sense, it is primarily concerned with relationships between shape, size, quantity and space. Dyslexic children often have difficulties with the basic computation skills involved in arithmetic and algebra. For instance, affected children may find it extremely hard to learn their times tables. Typically, they will begin chanting a table quite happily. Then they will lose their place, forget where they are and end up in a confused state reciting another table altogether. The following example illustrates this:

John recites the four times table

One times four is four,
Two times four is eight,
Three times four is twelve,
Four times four is sixteen,
Five times five — four — Is it four? — is — um— four— eight— no— twelve—? sixteen — sixteen!
Now where was I?
Four times five is twenty
Six times five is twenty four —No. That's not right.
Five times six is twenty-five.
What do you mean I'm supposed to be doing the four times not the six times? I'm hopeless.

This is meant to show that dyslexic children can easily lose the thread or sequence of what they are doing. Many of their parents are familiar with the difficulties that can be encountered with learning tables in the junior school, difficulties with the sequencing skills necessary for rapid and accurate recital of these tables and for other tasks which need rapid computation. Paradoxically, when dyslexic children reach the more advanced mathematical levels, they may well cope much better than other children and, in some instances, excel. The following genuine case study illustrates this:

Jenny

Jenny was a bright dyslexic child who struggled with mathematics throughout her primary and secondary schooling. However, although she lacked confidence completely in her own mathematical ability she nevertheless achieved a 'C' pass at GCSE mathematics through hard work and determination. She went onto university, where as part of her course, she was obliged to study modules in statistics and mathematics at degree level. Initially this caused a daunting and emotionally charged situation. Much counselling was required over long-distance telephone calls home to her father who had studied maths as part of his degree 30 years earlier. Unfortunately, he found he was not able to be of much help. Eventually, the student came home and a statistics tutor was found for her. In one afternoon he explained, in a way this student could understand, the basic concepts she needed to grasp. A month later she passed the statistics module examination with first class degree scores. This was because the advanced work she needed to cover for this course was easier for her than the basic arithmetic which had hindered her so greatly in the past.

This tendency for dyslexic children to fail on the tasks most other children find easy but shine on the more complex exercises is not restricted to mathematics. Dyslexic children are a little enigmatic at times. They appear to be poor at the easiest tasks and good at the hardest ones. If they can be nurtured through the problematic early stages, they will often blossom on more complex, sophisticated levels of study which require the higher-order, creative learning skills in which they often excel.

The following sections deal with a number of mathematical areas which often present particular problems for dyslexic children.

Self-Confidence

Self-esteem and self-confidence are central requirements for successful learners. This is especially true for Mathematics. Children may have a high anxiety level about the subject which has been subconsciously passed to them by parents who experienced similar problems. It may have been fostered by unsympathetic or inappropriate teaching. A negative self- image, lack of confidence and fear of failure are destructive influences on learning. They will compound children's difficulties and convince them that they will not succeed, that they are 'no good at maths'. It is often argued that mathematics is different from English. English is more about practising skills than mathematics, which constantly involves working at ever more complex concepts and calculations. As a result it can lead to more failure and more widespread failure.

It is therefore, essential, that every effort is taken to counter this potential for failure. The teaching methods which we recommend will assist by ensuring that children are given tasks which are within their competence, building on the maxim of success breeding success. More than this is required from the adults involved. At school marking will need to be sensitive and positive. A page of heavy red crossings out from the teacher with strongly critical remarks will not improve self-esteem. If a page of calculations is completely wrong the child needs an explanation as to how they can arrive at the right answer with some encouragement to persevere. Credit should be given for the calculations which are right or where the correct methods have been used even in they did not achieve the correct answer.

At home, children may well react emotionally to their perceived inability to complete homework successfully. Parents may feel emotional about that page of red crossings out and that strong remark. Home and school need to work together on this. If you are the teacher, arrange to see the parent and sort out a strategy for helping at home. If you are the parent, contact the school and arrange to see the teacher, to see how you can support the school. Do something positive.

Short-term Memory

Weak short-term memory can cause difficulties with mathematical sound–symbol correspondence. Mathematics has a code or language of its own. There is a relationship between the sign and the computation skill required. The sign '+' means 'add', the sign '×', that you multiply and so on. Children can become confused when trying to sort out which meanings go with each symbol, especially when they are busy trying to work out the calculation involved at the same time. To make it even more complicated, the word/words which relate to each symbol do not relate to a simple single word for each symbol. The following table indicates the number of synonyms for each of the **five key mathematical symbols**:

symbol	synonym
+	add, plus, increase, more than, the sum of, total
−	take away, minus, subtract, less than, difference between, decrease
=	means, equals, is, answer is, same as
÷	divide, share, split, give, how many, group
×	times, multiply, of, product of, power of

Each set of words in the previous table is a code word or synonym for the sign. Dyslexic children, who already have an acknowledged problem with information presented in the form of symbols, are therefore confronted with a twofold further complication. Firstly they can easily become mixed up between the function signs for adding, subtracting, multiplying and dividing. Secondly, they have to deal with the fact that these signs can be expressed in words with a number of synonymous alternatives. It is not surprising that they become confused.

In order to overcome this confusion, to help them accurately match the correct word with the correct symbol and the correct function with both, children will need much overlearning. For many children this is best achieved through a series of purposeful games and activities. We would recommend those designed by Anne Henderson which are included in the Resources Section at the end of the book.

A talking calculator can help here. The calculator immediately speaks the numbers and symbols which children have keyed in. This gives them a quick check on the accuracy of their perception of the calculation. (The technical term for this is that it gives an *'impartial auditory rehearsal'*.) What the calculator says has been keyed in may be quite different from what children intended or assumed they had keyed in. These calculators are cheap and available in high-street shops. We would recommend them for the dyslexic child who has significant difficulties with the discrimination of numbers and their recall.

Colour is a useful aid to assist distinguishing the correct symbol or word. As an example, all instances of addition might be in red, all division in blue and so on. Children could also be encouraged to construct a mind map to help clarify any confusions. This would contain the basic symbols and their associated words. Simple concrete examples could be incorporated so that they can see the whole and how the various parts relate to each other.

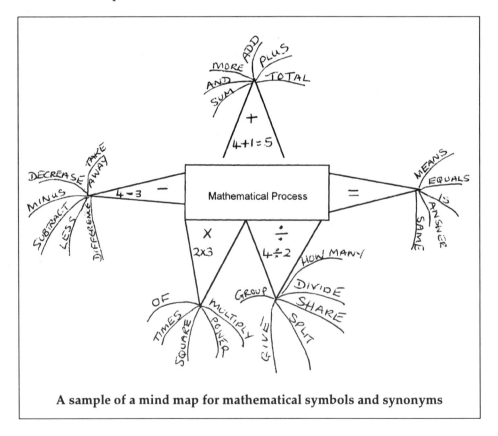

A sample of a mind map for mathematical symbols and synonyms

Direction and Orientation

Many dyslexic children have difficulties with direction and orientation which can affect their mathematical work. Frequently this occurs at the very simplest level where, when calculating, they forget from where they should start and in which direction to proceed. Reading and writing are always from left to right. This is not the case in mathematics. Look at these examples:

Addition is worked from right to left

L   46   ← Start this side   R

$$\begin{array}{r} 46 \\ + 50 \\ \hline 96 \end{array}$$

Subtraction is worked from right to left

L   36   ← Start this side   R

$$\begin{array}{r} 36 \\ - 22 \\ \hline 14 \end{array}$$

Multiplication is worked from right to left

L   15   ← Start this side   R

$$\begin{array}{r} 15 \\ \times\, 2 \\ \hline 30 \end{array}$$

But division is worked from left to right

L   Start this side   →   10   R

$$2\,\overline{)\,20}$$

As a consequence of these variations, dyslexic children have to remember not only the exact computation needed from the given sign, but also from where to start the sum and in which direction to work. No wonder we hear them say so often: *'Where do I start and which way do I go?'*

Orientation can also present difficulties, especially in the formation of figures and signs. The visual form of several numbers may easily be confused:

9 6   Mirror image

3 5   The direction of the top curve can easily be confused

3 8   These are often misread or miswritten as each other.

+ ×   These signs are actually the same but with a different orientation.

− +   Only the small dots distinguish these signs. Dyslexic children
             sometimes fail to notice or remember them.

Directional difficulties may also arise when children are asked to recall numbers in the correct sequence. For instance, 513 may be read as 315. This problem may be obvious at home with a child's inability to remember phone numbers in the correct sequence. It is caused by short-term memory weaknesses similar to those responsible for some spelling difficulties. The ability to recall a word visually, with the letters in the correct order, is just like that for numbers. However, the difference which a slightly wrong sequence of numbers can make to the outcome of a calculation is potentially more disastrous than a slightly wrong sequence of letters can make to understanding a sentence.

Example: The different consequences of poor visual recall on writing words and numbers

'The Pirme Minister calls on the Queen at Buckingham Palace each week.'

The reader will almost certainly work out what this writer meant by 'Pirme':

'The Prime Minister agreed to give £91,000,000 pounds to the Queen to refurbish her Palace.'

While the Queen may be content that this writer remembered the first two numbers in the wrong order, the Prime Minister would probably be rather upset.

Children can be helped to remember longer strings of numbers by encouraging them to chunk them in sub-sets. An example for a telephone number follows. The child is taught to learn them (in these chunks) giving each sub-set a rhythm so that it flows more easily:

Example: Breaking long numbers down into learnable chunks

01634   717964

01634   717   964

Accuracy in recalling and recording numbers sequentially is fundamental to successful computation.

Dyslexic pupils may have significant problems with place value or getting the decimal point in the correct place. These problems appear to be more related to difficulties with sequencing than in misunderstanding of the concepts involved.

Typically, they will simply recall or write the decimal point in the wrong place. 4.2 become 42, 3.678 becomes 36.78 and so on. Linked to this they will sometimes omit final '0's, so that, for instance, 400 becomes 40 or 4,000 is written as 4,00.

The net effects of these difficulties related to weak short-term memory, visual discrimination, sequencing and orientation may be to significantly affect a child's ability to calculate efficiently and accurately. We have shown that, in order to undertake some apparently simple calculations, **dyslexic children need to be competent in the following skills**:

- handle information presented in symbols; numbers and signs

- remember the form and function of each mathematical sign

- distinguish between similarly formed numbers and signs

- deal with the complexity caused by the large number of different synonyms for each sign

- understand and apply knowledge of the different directionality of different mathematical processes

These are all areas in which dyslexic children can have fundamental weaknesses. If they do it is no wonder that they should have difficulties with mathematical calculation.

The Inchworm and the Grasshopper

Three educational researchers, Bath, Chinn and Knox (see Booklist) identified two distinct types of mathematical learning style. The first is the quantitative style. This is related to an inchworm, a creature which moves to where it wishes to arrive slowly and methodically. The inchworm makes a step-by-step approach to mathematical problems, carefully following ground-rules and established methods of working things out. In contrast, there is the qualitative style of learning. This is likened this to a grasshopper. As its name implies, the grasshopper's style is very different. Frequently this kind of learner shows no sign of using a logical, orthodox approach to solving mathematical problems. There appears to be no methodology. Although to the grasshopper the approach used is logical, it is often bizarre and hard to follow.

Both these learning styles are acceptable and should be valid and valued in their own right. A grasshopper would not be the best person to audit a firm's accounts, but might be the best person to solve an otherwise insoluble problem by approaching it in a unorthodox way.

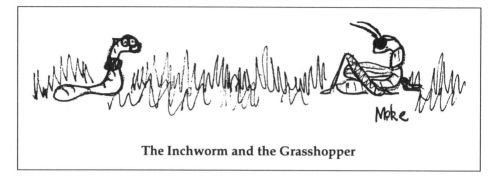

The Inchworm and the Grasshopper

While each learner's style should be valued for itself, problems can arise if the tutor and pupil are not in harmony with each other. An example of this can occur when an inchworm is being taught by a grasshopper or a grasshopper by an inchworm. You may not be surprised to learn that many dyslexic children are grasshoppers. Their mathematical workings often show quite different ways of thinking. They arrive at the same place as other children but via a markedly different route. The approaches which they use can be refreshing or perplexing, enlightening or frustrating. Although their methods and reasoning may be difficult to follow, they frequently work. They may well be using high-level mathematical thinking skills which are similar to those used for some great scientific and mathematical discoveries.

However, many teachers are inchworms. They are happiest using established methodology and practices which are efficient and effective but not always compatible with the grasshopper's way of thinking.

There is only one person who can change when a teacher's methods of teaching undermine or are incompatible with the learning style of the children. It cannot be the children. They will be unable to change in the radical way necessary. The onus must fall on the teacher who will need to make greater allowance for the children concerned. He or she must be prepared to mark positively for what may seem bizarre workings when the correct answer has been achieved. They must look for opportunities to praise and value children's unique learning style and to recognise their ability to see a problem from a different perspective. This does not mean accepting sloppy, rushed or ill thought-out work. It suggests that teachers should be prepared to look beneath the surface and acknowledge and praise children's positive achievements. This recognition should help give children the confidence needed to tackle what will probably be otherwise a difficult area for them.

Telling the Time

The relationship of time with space cause difficulties for some dyslexic children. These difficulties can persist even into the secondary stage. Some children appear to suffer from a kind of 'digital dissonance' or 'digital disability'. These are the ones who at the earliest age have been given a digital watch by parents or grandparents. These children are then encouraged to use the watch and given lots of practice. They chime out the numbers correctly on demand and the child gets instant success and feedback from it. This is fine as long as children are able to understand what the time is, what it means in relation to life and space and they are not relying merely on an ability to chant meaningless numbers on cue.

It may be better for the child to be given an analogue watch (traditional round dial), from the outset. With this kind of watch the child can actually see the time that is before and after the actual time shown and can begin to understand the meaning of time in relation to the space around.

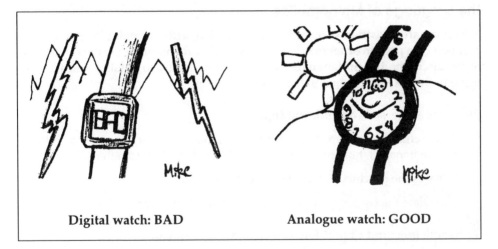

Digital watch: BAD   Analogue watch: GOOD

Encouraging use of an analogue watch is a useful strategy. Children using this type of watch from the outset, can see time in relation to their past and their future. They have a reference point and are able to use higher-level thinking skills to work out the relationship of time to their environment and life. It is not a meaningless jumble of numbers in isolation. If it is not seen in relation to time past and time future what does 3.42 actually mean?

We are not suggesting that learning to tell the time with an analogue watch will be easy. For instance, we cannot minimise all the associated problems of telling the time using 'past the hour' and 'to the hour'. But using a traditional watch face gives children an understanding of time which is not achievable through a digital watch. It is similar to the argument about using lap-top computers: if children have good keyboard skills and are struggling with getting their thoughts on to paper, then a lap-top will help them, especially in the short term. But it may also prevent them from ever being able to write effectively in their own hand. Perseverance with the more difficult skill — writing by hand — rather than giving up at the first obstacle can be far more beneficial in the long run. Children can switch to a digital watch or a lap-top when the basic concepts are learned and automatic. So if you are thinking of buying a watch for a Christmas or birthday present, we would recommend that you start at least with one which has the more traditional analogue face.

The ability to tell time accurately and manage time well will become increasingly important as children get older. Effective organisation of time is vital at secondary school. Many dyslexic children are not good organisers at this stage. We need, as educators and parents, to give our children strategies to help them understand and use time efficiently.

The Language of Mathematics

Mathematics is often seen as being concerned with an ability to manipulate numbers on a page in order to solve a problem. Clearly numbers are the key feature of this discipline, but the language of mathematics must also be taken into account. Some problems are couched in the form of writing:

Problems expressed in words not figures

'If one child had six apples, seven children had five oranges and ten children had no bananas, how many fruits would they have between them?'

'What is the product of seventeen and twenty four?'

'Calculate the square root of one hundred and forty four.'

To handle this kind of problem children must be able to:

- read and understand the text;

- handle sequentially a series of concepts;

- understand the terminology involved (e.g. product, calculate, square root);

- know how to solve the problem.

It can be seen that, in general, confronting dyslexic children with a written problem will tend to accentuate any underlying literacy difficulties. Their attempts to solve such problems will need careful structuring.

Alternatively children may be presented with problems which have not been written down in either numerical or word form. To some extent these non-verbal problems, usually referred to under the global term of mental arithmetic, can actually play to the strengths of dyslexic children. The attendant difficulties related to getting information from the written language are removed. Children are able to concentrate on the task itself without having to worry about extracting it from the page first. That said, the net effect of mental arithmetic may also be negative. The problem may well contain a series of tasks which children must retain in their working memory as they seek to first understand them, then decide the calculation tasks needed to solve it, then remember the figures to which the calculations which must be applied and then work out the answer. If the activity is timed (as it inevitably will be), children will then have to perform this sequence of tasks, which are intrinsically difficult for them, under extreme pressure. It is not surprising that, given this combined set of circumstances, some children become overloaded, stressed and give up. We have tried to illustrate this in the following example.

Example: 'Doing sums in my head or doing my head in'

(1) *The problem*

'If a drinking trough contains 60 litres of water work out how much is left after 6 cows have drunk 4 litres each, 10 litres have evaporated and the farmer has then re-filled it with 20 litres.'

(2) *Facts which need to be remembered*

- The trough starts with 60 litres.

- The cows drink 6 lots of 4 litres.

- 10 litres have evaporated.

- The farmer puts 20 litres more in.

(3) *The processes needed*

- I must first work out how much water left the trough.

- I must then take this away from 60.

- I must then add the 20 litres the farmer put in.

(4) *The skills needed*

- Remembering that 6 cows drank 4 litres each.

- Knowing that to work out the total of water drunk you must multiply 6 by 4.

- Being able to multiplying 6 x 4 in the head and get the right answer: 24

- Remembering that total.

- Remembering that 10 litres evaporated.

- Knowing that to work out how much water left the trough you must add the amount of evaporated water to the amount of drunk water.

- Being able to add 10 and 24 to get 34.

- Remembering that the tank had 60 litres to start with.

- Knowing that you must now subtract 34 from 60.

- Remembering that the answer is 26.

- Knowing that you must now add the 20 litres the farmer put in.

- Remembering that 26 litres are left.

- Knowing how to add 26 and 20 in your head.

- Not worrying that the rest of the class had their hands up 2 minutes ago to show they had finished and everyone is looking at you so that they can carry on.

- Knowing that the last time you did a similar problem you did not remember the numbers correctly and you got the sum wrong.

Maybe it is not surprising that some children give up in these circumstances, or fail even to try. If you do not try you cannot get it wrong. Maybe it is better to get told off for not appearing to care than humiliated because you do.

This potential difficulty for dyslexic children is worrying given the current move to incorporate mental arithmetic tests as part of formal National Curriculum and GCSE testing arrangements. As we have said before, for some children, non-verbal testing is advantageous. It allows them to show what they know without asking them to read or calculate on paper. For them it is essential not to judge their mathematical ability purely on tests which are based exclusively on decoding the written word. Non-verbal tests of mathematical ability, which concentrate on relationships between time and shape, size and quantity are more appropriate for assessing their mathematical functioning. Many of these pupils will rely on a calculator as an aid for the basic computation tasks. They may not have mastered their tables because of their weak-memory skills for figures in a sequence, but with the assistance of a calculator they can handle advanced mathematical problems with relative ease. If they cannot use a calculator for the new national tests they will be at a serious disadvantage. Special examination arrangements are needed which allow them to use calculators for mental arithmetic tasks. These should be fairly and consistently applied across the Boards. This would mean that dyslexic youngsters would not be further disadvantaged by their difficulties but enabled to show what they know. Surely it would not be improper for a calculator to be used in these circumstances? After all, what should be tested is the ability to apply mathematical principles to solve problems not the memory skills required to remember number patterns.

It is possible to be dyslexic and a good mathematician. Many dyslexics choose to take 'A' level mathematics and go on to study it at degree level. This is even after the experience of early difficulties which have been overcome with relevant tuition and the adoption of appropriate strategies. Usually not all areas of mathematics are affected. Some children will have an inherent weakness in only one specific area.

The use of technical aids (e.g. calculators) can be crucial. They should not be a substitute for children attempting to acquire proficiency in basic computation skills. However, when it is clear that lack of these skills, despite much effort, continues to hinder the further progress of children then use of a calculator, in particular, should be allowed and encouraged as a compensatory technique. It is paradoxical that within the normal mathematics curriculum, the higher the skill level of mathematics the more encouragement is given for all pupils to use technological aids. One only has to look at the quality of calculator required for 'A' level mathematics and the skill and competence needed to operate it compared to that for GCSE to demonstrate this point.

Using Mnemonics

Mnemonics can play an effective and efficient part in mathematics learning. The child who has difficulty in remembering formulae or equations can be encouraged to devise appropriate mnemonics to help memorise them. The illustration on the next page gives an example of a tried and tested mnemonic.

Using Key or Trigger Words

However, learning should not be by rote. What must be committed to memory needs, first and foremost, to be understood. Working out the reasoning behind a mathematical problem so that the correct computation can be identified is essential. Children should be taught to look for trigger words, signal words and key words. These will help them to concentrate on the key functions necessary for the calculation. They need to have the meanings of these key words very clear in their minds. The main words we have in mind follow. They are only a selection of mathematical words and certainly not an authoritative list.

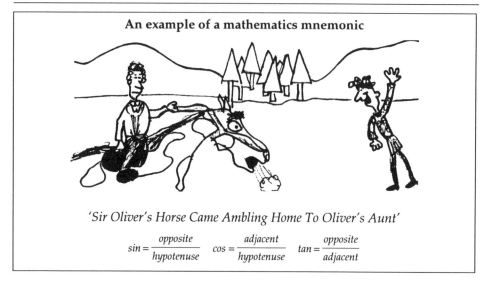

An example of a mathematics mnemonic

'Sir Oliver's Horse Came Ambling Home To Oliver's Aunt'

$$sin = \frac{opposite}{hypotenuse} \qquad cos = \frac{adjacent}{hypotenuse} \qquad tan = \frac{opposite}{adjacent}$$

Example: Key words and trigger words

addition   subtraction   division   multiplication   fraction   percentage

minus   times   plus   take   away   symmetry   perimeter

area   circle   decimal   angles   parallel   powers   roots   probability

Related to the need to be familiar with key words is the idea of collecting mathematical words within a mathematical dictionary. This will help ensure correct spelling and give an instant reference to the symbol /word and computation needed. Children should be encouraged to devise their own lists, appropriate to their needs and age group, in liaison with home or school. They can then group them as appropriate and illustrate the word with diagrams/captions/cartoons as the peg on which to hang the mathematical picture on to. The concept of thinking in pictures really does work for some dyslexic children. It can be extremely effective.

Some Concluding Thoughts

Many of the techniques that are used to alleviate literacy problems can be successfully transferred to those in mathematics. Multi-sensory teaching is essential, as are overlearning and revision. Mathematical teaching should be structured, sequential, cumulative and thorough. All of these recommendations, which the British Dyslexia Association makes for programmes of work on literacy, should be equally applicable for mathematics.

Teaching in a method appropriate to the way in which the child learns is as applicable in mathematics as it is in language learning. All the available channels to learning need to be utilised so that strengths are optimised and weaknesses reduced. If a child relies on a visual approach to learning and is weak with material presented through the hearing channel, then to teach entirely through an auditory approach would be unproductive. Far better to use all the channels so that the chance of building on a strength is maximised.

Children who feel that they have mathematical problems may become severely stressed when confronted with situations which threaten their security in this area. Common to most children who experience difficulties in this important subject is a distinct and often quite powerful lack of mathematical confidence. This may become almost a phobia, a 'mathephobia'. The use of mental arithmetic exercises in national testing will cause an increase in the anxiety levels of dyslexic children with mathematical difficulties. Anxiety, stress and panic are not conducive to a learning environment in which to build confidence in mathematics. Many dyslexics panic when faced with the restraints of examination conditions and time embargoes. It is to be hoped that a modern educational system will take account of this and recognise the needs of dyslexic pupils here, especially in regard to their real problems with short-term memory.

Assessment of mathematical ability should not be a test of memory skills. If a pupil knows and understands a mathematical concept and can apply it to work out a solution, then the fact that maybe their table bonds are weak or that simple computation is difficult without the aid of a calculator should not be an issue.

Finally, there are a number of excellent books written on dyslexia and mathematics which are included in the 'Resources section' later in this book. We recommend that you consult this section and use it as a basis for further investigation.

Summary of Chapter 6

This chapter

- gave an overview of dyslexia and mathematics;

- discussed factors which underlie good mathematical skills like short-term memory, self-confidence and orientation;

- showed how different children learn in different ways;

- discussed the language of mathematics;

- showed how mnemonics and using trigger words can help children learn.

Chapter 7

Dyslexia across the Curriculum

This chapter looks at the implications of being dyslexic for the whole of the
child's curriculum. It begins by looking at the processes involved in remembering and recalling information. It then describes a useful way of organising
information called mind-mapping. Other useful aids to memory are then covered. The effects of dyslexia on subjects across the curriculum are then
described. Children's visual and organisational skills are crucial in many subjects. These are discussed next. Finally, there is a guide to the jargon which
you may encounter in specialist reports written on these children.

Introduction

Memory difficulties have long been associated with dyslexia. The term
'short-term memory' frequently occurs in assessment reports prepared on dyslexic
children. What does this term actually mean? Short-term memory can be divided
into two broad areas: 'short-term visual memory'; and 'short-term auditory
memory'.

Some children are described as having a weak short-term visual memory when
they read or write. This means that they have difficulty in recalling the visual image
of the words they have seen. They have difficulty in retaining, in their memory, a
mental picture of what words look like. This leads to problems when they try to reproduce words accurately from memory. On the other hand, short-term auditory
memory refers to children's ability to hold strings of words or letters in their correct
sequence after they have heard them. It is linked to the skill needed to reproduce
these sequences accurately from memory when they write. Some dyslexic children
will have a weakness in one form of short-term memory and a strength in the other.
In severe cases, both forms will be affected.

Children need three linked skills when they wish to remember information.
These are the ability to see, store and recall accurately that information. Firstly, they
need to see or perceive the word precisely (*perception*). They must then store this information in the brain (*memory*). Finally they must be able to extract the information
from their memories when they wish to use it (*recall*). These three skills work together. They are hard to separate. Often, when we are asked for some information
we will say something like: 'It's there. I know it. It's on the tip of my tongue.' What
we mean when we say this is that we have heard or read this information before and

it is in our memory, but at that moment we cannot retrieve or recall it. For many dyslexic children, much of their reading and writing can be like this: a constant battle to perceive words correctly, memorise them precisely and recall them accurately. All three skills are essential for children to develop literacy and numeracy skills. Children with severe difficulties of perception, remembering and recall will need skilled and specific teaching to overcome them, usually focused on the multi-sensory methods we have emphasised in this book.

Our ability to process information in the memory is similar to the way computers function. For a computer to work effectively, information has to be inputted (perception) saved into its store of data (memory) and retrieved when it is needed (recall). Effective memory processing employs the same basic principles. Information is stored in the memory to be successfully recalled when it is needed. The diagram illustrates this process:

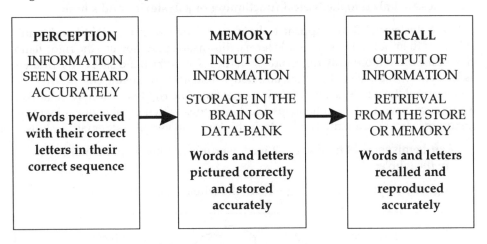

Perception, memory and recall

Dyslexics need to be taught explicit strategies for using their memories efficiently and for compensating for any weaknesses they may have.

Inputting of Information: Perception

The way information is inputted into memory is through the senses. These form pathways or channels which must be used fully if children are to process information effectively. All five senses may be used to strengthen and sharpen children's ability to perceive, store and recall information. By encouraging children to use all their senses, we increase the likelihood that information will be stored successfully in the memory. For example, some children are weak at remembering the visual images of words but strong in remembering their sound patterns. It would not be sensible to encourage continually these children to work mainly through their visual learning channels. The knowledgeable teacher will play to their strengths, but without ignoring the need to develop areas of weakness. The different senses should be worked together to underpin children's learning. They should be constantly linked and, wherever possible, used simultaneously. This is why multi-sensory teaching is so important.

Storage of Information: Memory

Once the information has flowed through the multi-sensory pathways into the memory, it must be stored so that it can be retrieved or recalled when necessary. This is often a difficult skill for dyslexic children. Once again though, teaching children appropriate strategies for storing information can be very worthwhile. These strategies are linked to the **typical functioning of a dyslexic child's brain.**

Some dyslexic children appear to be more in tune with the right-hand hemisphere of their brain. In very simple terms, this means that they use the right-hand side of the brain more fully for certain activities. The right-hand side of the brain is associated with the visual, spatial, and non-verbal activities using colour, rhythm, imagery and the whole as part of their processing. The right hemispherical thinker is less at ease with their left hemispherical functions which involve linear learning (learning in lines), sequential and orderly thinking and verbal mathematical skills.

Left-hemispherical thinking — Linear learning in lines — parts make up the whole;

Right-hemispherical thinking — Sees the whole from different angles.

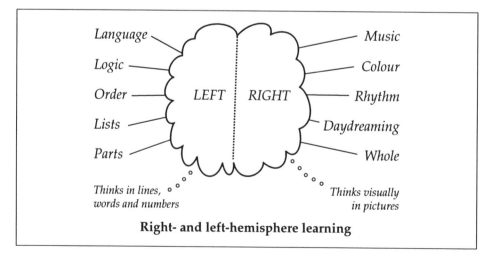

Right- and left-hemisphere learning

Mind-maps

As we wrote earlier in this chapter, one way of utilising the advantages of right-hemispherical thinking is to use the technique known as mind-mapping to help manage information (for more information on this we suggest you consult the excellent books by Tony Buzan — see Booklist). We have used several examples of mind-maps in previous chapters of this book. Mind-maps mainly use strengths which are located in right-sided thinking.

Attributes of mind-maps

- They use colour;

- They look at the global picture of a topic or theme;

- They clearly illustrate relationships between different aspects of the chosen subject;

- They encourage lateral thinking;

- They are based on using images and pictures.

Mind-maps can be used very effectively to plan and revise. They can also be used to make notes but we would suggest that this takes much more practice to become proficient.

The basic technique

(1) Children select the main image for the task they have to complete.

(2) This image is written and encircled at the centre of the map.

(3) Linked ideas and concepts are drawn within a series of satellites spread around this circle, to give a visual outline plan of all the main ideas and information they wish to include in their writing.

(4) The next stage is to concentrate on each of these satellites and identify ideas and facts linked to them and write them in a series of new, smaller satellites around the original ones.

The advantage of this method is that when children have completed the map, all the material they need for the assignment is visually summarised for them on a single sheet of paper. This is of great assistance to them in organising the material for their answer. It allows them to plan and structure each element into a logical and coherent sequence which develops the main theme. As we have stressed throughout this book, dyslexic children often have difficulty in organising their thoughts in this way. Mind-mapping helps them to do so. When children have spent time planning their work in this way, they can then concentrate on getting their ideas over to the reader in a lively and original way. If they had to continually worry about getting these ideas down logically, their creative ability would be correspondingly reduced.

You have seen how this can work already in the example we gave in Chapter 5 of a mind-map based on the title 'My Kitchen' as a theme for an essay. If you look back you will see that this mind-map began with the central theme 'kitchen' encircled at the centre of the plan. The child then chose a series of sub-headings related to the kitchen she wished to describe. When this was completed further sub-headings were added. With this plan firmly in her mind, the writer was then able to concentrate on developing it on paper in the language she needed to highlight her theme. Freed from the need to simultaneously structure her answer, she was enabled to produce an attractive, affectionate and wry response which might otherwise have been impossible for her. A further example of making a mind-map follows:

Making a mind-map

(1) This is very easy to do. Imagine children have been set the following assignment for their English course question.

Using the book to help you, write a 'Who's who' about each of the characters in 'Carrie's War'. Your answer should include the following:

(a)   a detailed description of what they look like (appearance)

(b)   their relationships with the other characters in the book

(c)   their personality as people

Use evidence from the book to support your answer.

Using the mind-map technique to plan this task, children must first decide the central theme. They would probably choose the main characters in this book, Carrie and her brother Nick. This would be the central image. It does not need to be a work of art. There is no need to be good at drawing to successfully mind-map. Stick people can say as much as detailed figures. It must however be meaningful and trigger the whole concept. The central image chosen is of two figures with labels around their necks within the letter C.

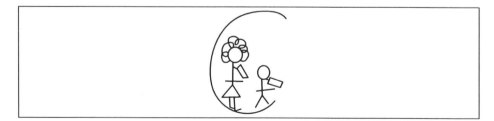

(2) From this central image radiate the main themes in different colours. A single
     word — a key word — is chosen that unlocks the meaning and this is written in
     block capitals on each strand or theme. In this case it will be the characters.

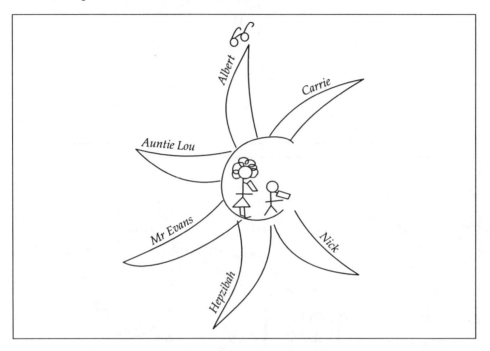

   One of the main advantages of using mind-maps with dyslexic children is that
they can immediately see the whole picture and the overview of the characters in
the book. By keeping the colours related to individual characters the same, there is
an immediate grouping of details concerning that character. This helps to retain
that information in the memory. Another advantage of planning using this system
is the ability to add on at a later date, without needing to start again. This keeps the
cohesion intact and gives children the flexibility to develop their response further
without hindering the sequence. The method actually aids sequencing. When the
mind-map is complete, each section can be numbered and written out in the order
of the whole. The child or adult can see what is to go first, what then follows and
how the assignment can be planned from character to character.

   The next diagram shows a mind-map of the main themes from the book 'Of Mice
and Men' by John Steinbeck. This mind-map is not complete but it does show the
central image and the main themes of the book radiating from it. It now needs the
detail put in.

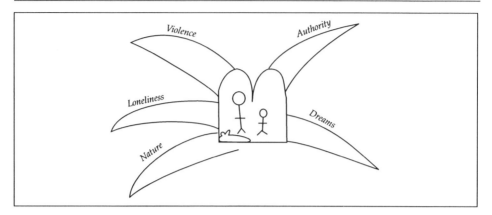

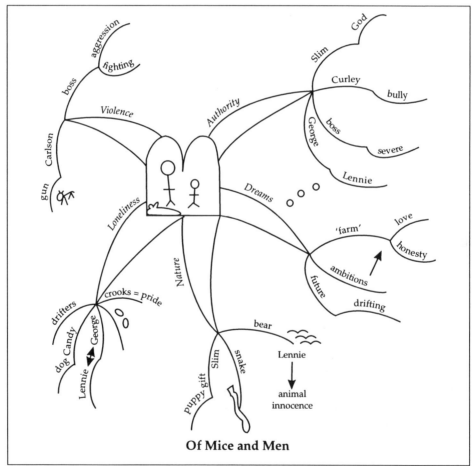

Of Mice and Men

From experience in teaching severely dyslexic pupils, one of the most frequently heard comments is: *'What do you mean by revision? How do you revise?'* Mind-mapping is a useful technique for revision. It is time-consuming but it does work. The act of making a mind-map is a form of revision in itself. Choosing keywords is a skill which relies on understanding concepts and applying knowledge (e.g. to make a mind-map in geography on volcanoes needs a basic understanding of what volcanoes are). Keywords will therefore reinforce children's real grasp of the subject. It will instil knowledge into the memory far more effectively than the mindless repetition of lists of facts or the aimless reading which many children believe is revision.

You may have noticed a resemblance between mind-mapping and a similar method called brainstorming. However, it is only a resemblance. In brainstorming, the information is put down in random order. There is little emphasis on structure . Mind-mapping relies on grouping information in a recognised way, based on colour, themes and images. Once the technique has been taught and applied, children will hopefully learn to value its use because it will help them to be more successful. This will encourage them to persevere with it until it becomes a habit. It can then be applied with ease, and become an automatic and preferred way of thinking and planning. Children may find it strange to begin with, but as with most skills, with practice they will become adept and confident at this form of planning and revision which builds on the strengths of many dyslexics.

Mind-mapping can be used for virtually all subjects and for all levels of learning. It is not restricted to schools but can be equally applicable to university. A dyslexic student known to one of the authors uses this technique for all revision at university, to valuable effect.

Completed mind-maps should not be discarded. When complete, a mind-map has only fulfilled half of its task. The other half is to use it to revise, putting that essential information into the memory in such a way that it can be quickly retrieved when needed. The actual size of paper used is not very important but we would recommend that children start with A3 paper, (about the size of a broadsheet newspaper). If the chosen paper proves to be too small, then extra sheets can be cellotaped on to it. One of the most successful mind-maps we have seen took over the walls of a sixth form student's bedroom. When complete, the student took 5 or 10 minutes every night to review and trace certain aspects of the mind-map that she needed to revise. To her parents it did not seem to make much sense. They understood it was all about 'Business Studies', but could not follow its complex patterns of images and colours, crossings-out and connecting lines. This often happens. Mind-maps are personal. Often they only mean something to the people who have made them. We have shorthand ways of recording things which do not involve writing words. For example, except for cheques, we rarely write the word *'pounds'*. Usually writing the sign '£' is enough to convey the correct meaning.

There are some dyslexic children who have been taught mind-mapping techniques but do not use them. They may not see them as relevant to their needs. This should be respected. Children should not be forced to use a method with which they are not happy. What we suggest is that they are taught how to mind-map and encouraged to give the technique a reasonable chance before they either discard or adopt it. Incidentally one of the authors now uses this technique for all planning at work and this book was originally planned using a mind-map.

Mnemonics

There are other memory aids which are relevant. As mentioned in the chapter on spelling, the use of mnemonics is commonplace and a very good way of remembering easily confused signs or sequences. For example, in Science, the colours of the rainbow can be remembered by the picture and sentence:

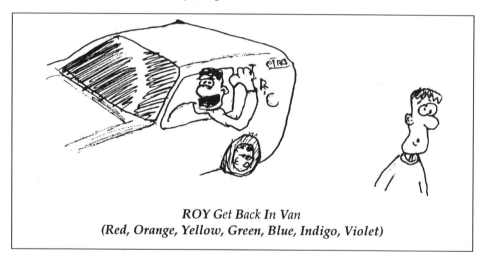

ROY Get Back In Van
(Red, Orange, Yellow, Green, Blue, Indigo, Violet)

There are many individual variations on this which are all applicable as long as they are remembered.

Some useful spelling mnemonics

(1)   A **pie**ce of **pie**. *(To remember the difficult 'pie' sequence in 'piece'.)*

(2)   Never be**lie**ve a **lie**. *(The same thing with the 'lie' sequence here.)*

(3)   Ne**c**essary has one **c**ollar and **two s**ocks. *(There is one 'c' and two 'ss'.)*

(4)   A spe**cia**l agent is someone in the **CIA**. *(The 'cia' sequence in 'special'.)*

(5)   A **bus** is **bus**y — good business. *(A reminder that 'busy' spelt with a 'u' not an 'i'.)*

(6)   It's **great** to **eat**. *(To help children remember how to spell that 'eat' sequence.)*

(7)   **You** are **you**ng. *(Similarly with 'you' in 'young'.)*

(8)   **Big Elephants Can't Always Use Small Exits.** *(To help remember 'because'.)*

(9)   You'll need a **drain** for the **rain**. *(To help remember that 'ain' sound.)*

(10)   A **U** turn. *(To remember it's 'u' although it may not sound like it.)*

(11)   It **it**ches. *(The 't' is not obvious. This will help remind children about it.)*

(12)   An **island is land** surrounded by water. *(That silent 's' catches many.)*

(13)   **Cat**ch a **cat**. *(As does the hard to hear 't' in 'tch' sequences.)*

(14)   **Committee — 2ms, 2ts, 2es —** 1 Chairman/8 members. *(Self-explanatory.)*

(15)   **Unusual —** unusual word with **3 u's**. *(Self-explanatory.)*

(16)   **U** and **I** build a house. *(The silent 'u' catches many. This may help.)*

(17)   Magic **Ian** is a magic**ian**. *(Should help recall of this difficult ending.)*

(18)   **Laugh —** Lions And Unicorns Go HaHaHa *(Strong, funny image to fix in mind.)*

(19)   **O U** lucky duck sh**ould**, c**ould**, w**ould**. *(Same again.)*

Chunking

Children can improve their memory for information by chunking it. In Chapter 5 we illustrated this with the image of eating a bar of chocolate. The image was intended to show how much easier it is to handle and enjoy information (and chocolate) when it is broken down into chunks or slabs. The same analogy works with memory . We find it easier to remember information when it is chunked into *'bite-sized'* pieces. A good example of this is the way we remember telephone numbers. Most people tend to automatically chunk these numbers into groups of three or four. They do this because it is easier to remember them that way. This is easily demonstrated.

Which is harder to remember?

0124763886   or   0124 763 886?

We would expect readers to find the unbroken string of numbers '0124763886' harder to remember than the chunked sequence of '0124 – 763 – 886.' This principle can be applied to spelling or indeed any piece of information that needs to be remembered. Effective spelling programmes build on this principle. In chapter 3 (spelling) we referred to lists of different letter strings which are taught in groups. Using this method children are taught common letter sequences in families. Examples are: *'str'*, *'ear'*, *'tion'* and *'con'*. One of the key reasons for doing this is to encourage children to build up their memory for these basic spelling sequences by presenting them in chunks, with the intention that this will assist their retention in the memory.

Rhyme

Another way of fixing information in the memory is to use rhyme and rhythm. The work of two reading specialists Lynette Bradley and Peter Bryant (see Booklist) has shown that children's familiarity with, and ability to recognise and use basic rhymes, is vital to the development of literacy skills. They found that children whose parents had read and sung nursery rhymes to them learnt to read more quickly and easily.

This facility with rhymes will have uses later in another way, when simple rhymes can be used to help instil information in the memory. For example, we all know most of Henry VIII's wives did not live to a ripe old age but few of us could easily say how they met their separate fates. Yet this simple, rather stark little verse could impressively improve our memory, at a stroke you might say:

Henry's wives' lives

Divorced, beheaded, died;
Divorced, beheaded, survived.

Most of us remember the fate of Guy Fawkes with this little rhyme:

Remember, remember, the fifth of November
Gunpowder, treason and plot.

Obviously new rhymes cannot be dreamt up for every piece of information which a child needs to learn. However, most children will develop blocks about learning certain fundamental pieces of information. Building that information into a simple and striking rhyme will help them remember it.

Planning Revision Time

It is important that children use their memories fully. As we stated earlier, if there is a weakness in one sensory channel then it makes sense not to be dependent on that channel as the means of input or retrieval of information. However, it is not enough merely to input information into the memory and expect it to be retrieved on demand without revision. Other more subtle influences are at work. For instance, common sense might tell you that children will remember facts most efficiently in the middle of a revision session rather than at either end. You might logically assume that, at the beginning, they will not have got going, and at the end they will be too tired. The reverse seems to be true. Research has shown that we remember the beginning and ending of a period of study time more effectively than the middle section. If this is the case then it would make sense when children plan their revision, to build in frequent breaks to increase the number of separate sessions. This will ensure more beginnings and endings and therefore more effective input into the memory. In this context, we would recommend that for older children, perhaps revising for GCSE, a period of study time becomes unproductive after about an hour. A break is needed at that point. Children should be encouraged to stop for 10 to 15 minutes, perhaps doing something completely different. When they return to their studies at the end of this break, their learning will be the more efficient for it.

The Effects of Dyslexia on Individual School Subjects

One of the themes of this book is that dyslexia is far more than a reading difficulty. It often affects children's performance in many areas of the school curriculum. The next section of this chapter describes the kinds of difficulty which the condition may give rise to in different curriculum areas. This is not to say that all dyslexic children will have these difficulties. Whether they do or not will vary according to the specific nature of children's dyslexia and the way the subject is taught. There could be unexpected problems in curriculum areas which would not usually be associated with dyslexia.

Access to the Curriculum

You may have heard the phrase 'access to the curriculum' being used about children with special educational needs. This phrase refers to how accessible a subject is to the children who are taking it. The accessibility of a subject is an important factor in the capacity of dyslexic children to perform well within it, to understand it and to show their understanding. Accessibility relates to the demands subjects place upon children. Factors which decrease accessibility for dyslexic children are easy to identify. In general those lessons which require children to read and write frequently will be harder to access than practically based lessons. If reading and writing are an essential part of a lesson, the way in which the teacher handles that requirement will also affect its accessibility. For instance, if teachers expect children to read books whose text is too difficult for them or to write at greater length or complexity than they are capable of, then their lessons will be largely inaccessible to them. If, on the other hand, extra help is available to assist them with difficult text, or the teacher will allow them to answer a question in note form or orally, then the subject will be much more accessible. Giving children access to the curriculum, therefore, is another way of saying that it is appropriate to their needs or has been adapted to meet their needs.

Dyslexia and Language Skills

It is with language skills that most difficulties would be anticipated. The ability to read is immediately to the fore. However, some dyslexic children do not have reading difficulties or have improved their reading skills to such an extent they no longer present a problem. An inability to spell quickly and accurately is more predictably a major problem with English as a subject.

English involves more than the ability to read and write. Children's skill in understanding what is said to them (receptive language) and communicating their thoughts and feelings in speech (expressive language) are fundamental to the English curriculum. Dyslexic children may have difficulties with both expressive and receptive language. We have mentioned before the problems some dyslexic children have in 'naming', in finding the right word to express their meaning. They know the word they need, they know they know it, but they cannot find it quickly enough in their personal store of words. Or when they do find it, they get it all muddled up or back to front.

A dyslexic pupil approached the teacher complaining about the sore inside his mouth:

> Miss, I've got one of those things in my mouth. Oh! What are they called? You know what I mean, those, those bumgoils.

This kind of expressive language difficulty can be time-consuming and frustrating for parents, teachers and children. However, children will usually find the word needed or, in some cases, be skilled in inserting another word which is similar in meaning to the one wanted. It is astonishing to experience the skill some dyslexic children have in finding alternative words with the same meaning as the one they cannot remember. However, it will not be the word they wanted and may be an inferior word. Imagine if Shakespeare had had a word-finding problem. He may have written: 'A pony, a pony, my kingdom for a pony!' rather then his strikingly original cry for a horse.

This reflects the danger that, in successfully finding an appropriate word, children may impair the quality of their work by choosing a safe but ordinary alternative to the more vivid or dramatic word of their preferred choice. A similar phenomenon can be found in some dyslexic children's writing when they choose safe easy-to-spell words rather than the more complex and appropriate vocabulary they would prefer to use if they were confident they could spell it accurately.

Children with receptive language difficulties may have difficulties in retaining information in their working memory. They may not be able to understand and follow sentences which contain complicated or lengthy information. This can lead to acute problems when the teacher is giving them instructions. If children do have problems in this area, it is important that teachers are aware of it. If not, they may unwittingly ask more of children than they are able to give. For instance, take this not uncommon scenario, when the teacher instructs children in the homework required of them:

> Well done. Good lesson. Don't close your books yet. For homework I want you to find Exercise 3 on page 57. Can you finish the first six sums please and then all of Exercise 4? Got that? Right. It's Thursday's homework so bring it in for Friday's lesson. Off you go.

This is not an exaggerated example. It reflects the instruction given out by many teachers at the end of a busy lesson, with the next group already starting to queue up outside. It is likely that dyslexic children with receptive language difficulties will only be able to remember two or three separate elements in their working memory at one time.

From this example, they might remember the following:

- Homework has been set;

- It's in the class textbook;

- It was on page fifty something.

The teacher should not be surprised if the child does not actually do the homework in time or does Exercise 7 on page 53 for the following Thursday. One county tries to anticipate this difficulty by recommending for all secondary dyslexic children that each teacher should:

> ... ensure that the child understands the homework to be done and has written it down accurately.

If they have difficulties in this area, children should have instructions limited to two or three elements at the most. Ideally, in this context, the teacher in the example might have written the homework on the board previously, have stopped the class with a few minutes to go, have pointed to the blackboard and said:

> Write down your homework. In by Friday, please.

This would have been so much more accessible to any dyslexic child in the class. If it is inevitable that instructions will contain several elements, then the teacher should space them. One or two instructions should be given first, with a pause for children to follow them. Other elements should be added at a reasonable pace. The homework given might have been introduced like this:

> Open your books to page 57. Have you found it?
> *Pause*
> Good. Find Exercise 3.
> *Pause*
> You have to answer the first 6 questions.
> *Pause*
> When you have finished those, answer Exercise 4 please.
> *Pause*
> In by next Friday.

It helps to reinforce oral instructions by writing them on the board or overhead projector. When they have been written, the teacher could then repeat them orally, pointing to them as this is done. It may seem a little laborious, but one spin-off could be that all the children fully understand what they have to do. This will save a lot of individual questions later. If the teacher has the time, any dyslexic children could then be asked to say the instructions aloud. This will help to clarify what children are to do. If it sounds like multi-sensory teaching (saying, as you read, as you point) then that is intentional.

The power of language cannot be underestimated for all children and especially for dyslexic children. As the Kingman Report stated at the start of the National Curriculum in 1988:

> Language expresses identity, enables co -operation, and confers freedom. In language we create a symbolic model of the world, in which past and present are carried forward into the future. Language is the naming of experience and what we name we have power over.

Dyslexia and Mathematics

Mathematics has a language of its own, its own code. If children are denied access to the key to this code they cannot break it. For example a problem may be expressed entirely in words, without a single number or symbol. Dyslexic children who are non-readers or weak readers may not be able to solve it even if they know the processes involved to do so. If the problem had been expressed in numbers they might have been able to successfully complete it. Similarly problems will arise if children muddle a mathematical sign with the function it represents: there will be limited or no success.

Dyslexia and Science

This is traditionally an area of strength for dyslexic children, but it still has some problem areas. The most obvious of these is the frequent need to read text which may be quite complex and may use difficult, unfamiliar words. Some schools will help dyslexic children here by preparing them to read new vocabulary before it is introduced to the mainstream class.

A difficulty specific to science is the need for many experiments to be written up in a precise sequence: the order in which they occurred in the experiment. This can be a very difficult task for dyslexic children who have weak sequencing skills. It will be compounded if the teacher requires the experiment to be written up for homework. It is not surprising that many dyslexic children have such homework returned from the teacher with comments like:

You tried hard but it was too muddled for me to follow it properly.

If children could respond to their teachers this pupil may have written:

I understood the experiment and I wanted to do well but you didn't give me a proper chance.

A further complexity is that science has its own language and, in some instances, its own sound–symbol matching. The periodic table is a good example where the names of elements are matched with their symbols. This has the potential to be confusing for dyslexic children.

Dyslexia and Music

Music also has its own language or code. This literally involves matching sounds with symbols. In addition it has an extra dimension with the naming of notes and rhythm, pitch and time. This is not to say that dyslexic children will find music inaccessible. The reverse seems to be true for many of them. The authors have personal experience of two dyslexic children who not only managed to successfully play musical instruments but who also gained good examination grades in music. There are many examples of successful musicians who are also dyslexic. The Associate Board examinations take the needs of dyslexic candidates seriously when they are sitting their music examinations. This is not a concession. It is designed to give dyslexic musicians an opportunity to sit these exams without being unnecessarily hindered by their dyslexia (see the Booklist).

Dyslexia and Modern Foreign Languages

Recent research from America, comparing good and weak foreign language learners, has indicated that the weaker learners tend to have less well developed phonological skills (weak at matching sounds with symbols). This is a known weakness of many dyslexic children. It seems to follow that if these children are experiencing difficulties in matching sound and symbol in their own language, then the additional burden of learning another language which has a different sound–symbol code, could lead to undue pressure, confusion and overloading.

'But I can't spell in English, let alone in French' is a common plea from failing and struggling dyslexic children. The source of their struggle is easily identifiable. There are a number of skills which are crucial when learning a foreign language: — sound–symbol matching, short-term memory and naming ability — that are known weaknesses for dyslexics. The skills are central to the subject and must be very familiar to our readers by now. This is not to say that all dyslexic children should be denied the opportunity to learn a foreign language. Many do so successfully. Most will enjoy the experience of learning a new language, especially if it is taught to them appropriately, ideally using a multi-sensory approach.

Languages which have a regular phonetic structure and pronunciation such as German, Spanish and Welsh are probably easier for dyslexic children to learn. School administrators and teachers should take this into account when time-tabling and making curriculum choices. Some researchers believe that it is not appropriate to choose French as modern foreign language for dyslexic children to learn because of its unfamiliar phonic structure and pronunciation.

Dyslexia and Humanities

The term 'humanities' embraces history, geography and religious education. Each of these subjects can present specific difficulties for dyslexic children. For instance in geography, there may be problems with the directional skills and sound–symbol relationships necessary for map-reading and using grid references.

History might present difficulties for a dyslexic when faced with chronology and the identification of historical events in relation to time. Matching an historical event to a specific date is a similar activity to matching a sound with its symbol. History will often require good reading ability especially when it requires the higher-order reading skills necessary to extract information from source material.

Dyslexia and Physical Education

Traditionally PE would not be associated with dyslexic-type difficulties. However, many dyslexic children will have accompanying problems with either fine (small movements) or gross (large movements) motor skills. Not unexpectedly PE requires these skills to a relatively high degree. The subject also emphasises balance and hand-to-eye coordination, another area of development which can place some dyslexic children at a distinct disadvantage. There are many dyslexic children who are not 'naturals' at ball games. As a result of their apparent clumsiness and poor co-ordination, they will be the ones automatically left at the back of the line when teams are being chosen. The type of poor motor control or clumsiness to which we are referring may be due to a number of factors or a combination of them. The **underlying causes of poor motor control or clumsiness** are:

(a) general poor coordination

(b) low muscle control

(c) weak balance

(d) left/right confusion

(e) lack of body awareness

(f) poor spatial awareness

(g) a poor sense of direction

(h) weak auditory memory

(i) poor sequencing skills

(j) weak ball skills and an inability to forecast velocity

(k) underdeveloped extended arm skills

Children who are affected in these ways may be reluctant to use space and will not attempt activities or movements which they consider risky. Many dyspraxic (see Glossary) children fall into this category.

However, there are many examples of outstanding sports people who are also dyslexico, for example, Duncan Goodhew, the swimmer and Steven Redgrave, the Olympic oarsman. Many dyslexic children represent their schools in a variety of sports. The message here is: do not despair if children lack proficiency at traditional school games. Try other sports. Water sports are a good example: sailing, wind surfing, rowing and canoeing are great fun, very competitive and require skill and strength.

Dyslexia and Art

This is a common area of excellence for dyslexic children. Many art teachers are surprised to discover that the child they meet in their weekly art lesson who shows such flair, imagination, creativity and talent may be described in very different ways by colleagues in other areas of the curriculum. If dyslexia is a specific learning difficulty in most subjects, then in the context of art it can be seen as a specific learning strength. The term 'dyslexia' does not present a uniform negative picture across the curriculum.

Dyslexia and Technology

Technology is another area where dyslexics may excel. This is connected to their strengths in right-hemispherical thinking skills. Technology is a broadly based subject with many sub-groupings: textiles, graphics, food technology, design, pottery, metalwork, woodwork and plastics. It does not necessarily follow that children will be talented in all of these areas, simply because they are dyslexic. What we are saying is that they may have a particular strength in one or more of these areas and it should be recognised and valued.

Dyslexia and Information Communication Technology (ICT)

This is another skill area of the curriculum where many dyslexics can display their potential and their high-level reasoning skills. To some extent, ICT can release that straitjacket imposed by poor literacy skills which hampers many dyslexia children. The use of the computer to solve problems, to present material in way that is visually acceptable and valued by society gives them greater freedom than pen and ink alone.

In North America, and to a lesser extent in the United Kingdom, there is now a trend for employers to actually prefer to engage bright, dyslexic applicants who are computer literate. These people are more likely to see the global picture necessary for this area of work, to produce a new and fresh view of the product concerned.

We are in the midst of a technological revolution equivalent to the industrial revolution. The key exponents of this new technology will benefit from the talent to perceive the world in a different way. People who have strengths in high-level thinking skills, especially many of those which are right hemispherical in origin, will be in demand. These skills will be valued and demanded by this new society in preference to the exclusive ability to read and write well.

Dyslexia and Organisation

When entering a new school, whether it is the first time in the infant class, the junior school or at the secondary stage, most children experience difficulty in adjusting to the new demands made on them. These demands are mainly caused by factors outside of their control. Many of these will be inherent in the school environment or the curriculum. They are concerned with the structure of the school and its size, its procedures, its personnel and its expectations of its pupils. The complexity of school life which these facets represent can confront dyslexic children with a number of very real challenges. This section looks at those challenges and suggests how children may be assisted to meet them.

Transferring between primary and secondary school

Many children find transferring from junior school to secondary school a daunting experience. Dyslexic children arrive at secondary school facing the same difficulties as other children, but with the added disadvantage of their often weak organisational skills. For instance, they will have to remember the names of their different teachers, what they teach, when they teach it and what room it is taught in. Then they must remember which lessons are on which days, where to go for each lesson and what books and equipment are needed. They must then remember what homework has been set and when it should be handed in. Some children will need to bring dinner money and many must also learn to always carry their bus pass along with the Homework Diary and the money that was borrowed from Reception yesterday because the dinner money was forgotten.

For the majority of the school's new pupils, these routines and facts will be quickly learnt. However, for dyslexic children, the whole experience can initially seem confusing and bewildering, even overwhelming. If children still have difficulty remembering whether Thursday is before or after Tuesday or they cannot sequence the months of the year, their sense of time can become inconsequential and confused. If these same children do not have a watch or cannot tell the time, organising life around a time-table presents them with major problems. They may become very muddled, perhaps forgetting whether bells mean the end of one lesson or the beginning of another, perhaps losing things and leaving possessions in forgotten places. It is no wonder that they can become distressed and frustrated. This potential for disorientation and distress will have repercussions which the teaching staff and parents will need to manage carefully and sympathetically.

Planning the week ahead

Many schools use an individual weekly planner to help. This will assist them to organise themselves each day before they leave home for school. A typical planner is reproduced in the table below. Usually it will be firmly affixed to the inside flap of their school bag or displayed prominently in their bedroom or the kitchen. Especially in the early stages, parents will usually be asked to check that their child has consulted the planner before they leave for school.

An example of a planner

Day	Bring/do	Homework
Monday	Dinner money Homework diary signed	Maths Science
Tuesday	Swimming money Swimming costume, goggles and towel	English French
Wednesday	Cooking ingredients	Maths Humanities
Thursday	PE kit	English Welsh
Friday	Holiday money	Science

Dyslexic children tend to lose equipment and clothing more frequently than most of their classmates. Marking clothing discreetly with their names will help here.

Organising writing and recording

There are other organisational features besides time and management. Some dyslexics have difficulties dealing with the actual space on the page and their writing on it. If instructions are given in a clear, logical and concise way, they will have a much better chance of producing neat work because they know exactly what is required of them. Structure can be built onto the page through a type of scaffolding approach where initially the parent or teacher will draw boundaries for the child to work within, gradually extending these, paralleling them with the level of success obtained, until the child is working freely on the whole page with confidence and organisation. They will need rules and routines reinforced and made very explicit to them. Teachers and parents need to be firm. They should insist, for instance, that all titles and headings should be underlined and the underlining should be made with a ruler. Instructions to do so should be made very clear and explicit. A good way of ascertaining whether children have understood what is required is to ask them to explain to you what they need to do. This is another instance of auditory rehearsal. It will reinforce in children's minds the processes which have been laid down. It will also double-check their understanding of the expectations which are being made for them.

Getting to know you

Thomson and Watkins (see Booklist) suggest that teachers should go through three distinct phases in their relationships with their dyslexic pupils. Initially there will be an 'earthing' period. At this stage they will be accepted by the teacher in a non-judgemental way. They will be welcomed by them into the class. At this first stage the teacher and parent do all the organisation for the children, giving them a chance to settle in, relax and be themselves.

When children are established, comfortable and ready to accept more responsibility themselves, the second stage begins. This involves the teacher and parent reducing their input until they are directly assisting for about 50% of the time. In doing so the aim is for children to learn to organise themselves supported by a responsible adult. Finally there is the 'challenging ' phase. This is when the adults gradually withdraw their support until the point is reached where children will organise themselves automatically.

Dyslexic children will often take longer to complete tasks and may have to work much harder than their peers to produce work of the same quality. They will not appreciate doing unnecessary work or the wrong task. Concentration levels and tiredness thresholds can be reached much sooner because children incorrectly interpreted the task required.

On the following pages you will find two prompt sheets which have been designed to help children and teachers get organised. The first one is a prompt for the child to fill in each night from Sunday to Thursday nights. The second is an organisational overview prompt for busy teachers and parents. It is designed give the teacher a quick visual check on individual children's organisational progress and needs.

CONFIDENTIAL

SCHOOL	INDIVIDUAL ORGANISATION CHECKLIST

PUPIL	TUTOR GROUP	DATE

This checklist is designed to help you. Please fill it in using your timetable to help you. You must check every night that you have included all the things you need for next day in your bag when you pack it . Do not leave this important task to the morning when you are rushed for time. Do it before you go to bed. Put this list on your bedroom wall.

SUNDAY NIGHT   CHECK THAT HOMEWORK HAS BEEN DONE
Pen, pencils, rubber, calculator, ruler, pencil case, homework diary,

MONDAY NIGHT   CHECK THAT HOMEWORK HAS BEEN DONE
Pen, pencils, rubber, calculator, ruler, pencil case, homework diary,

TUESDAY NIGHT   CHECK THAT HOMEWORK HAS BEEN DONE
Pen, pencils, rubber, calculator, ruler, pencil case, homework diary,

WEDNESDAY NIGHT   CHECK THAT HOMEWORK HAS BEEN DONE
Pen, pencils, rubber, calculator, ruler, pencil case, homework diary,

THURSDAY NIGHT   CHECK THAT HOMEWORK HAS BEEN DONE
Pen, pencils, rubber, calculator, ruler, pencil case, homework diary,

HAVE YOU REMEMBERED YOUR HOMEWORK DIARY AND HOMEWORK?

CONFIDENTIAL

	INDIVIDUAL EDUCATION PLAN ORGANISATION
SCHOOL	

PUPIL	YEAR	DATE

ASSESSMENT **TEACHER**
FACULTY/ PASTORAL

H SECTION	YES	WORKING	NO
1. HOMEWORK			
Completes homework			
Hands homework in			
Meets homework deadlines			
2. DIARY			
Has a homework diary in school every day			
Sets out the homework diary fully			
Records homework in the homework diary			
Gives the diary to parents/guardians to sign			

P SECTION	YES	WORKING	NO
1. PUNCTUALITY			
Is punctual for school			
Is punctual for lessons			
2. EQUIPMENT			
Brings appropriate kit/equipment for lessons			
calculator, PE kit, Technology, pencil/pens/ ruler			
3. BOOKS			
Has appropriate exercise book/file for lesson			
Has appropriate textbook/ worksheets/ maps etc			
4 .COURSEWORK / PROJECT			
Completes coursework /project			
Meets deadline for coursework / project			
Works to best of ability in coursework and projects			

TARGETS **DATE**

1.

2.

FURTHER ADVICE IS AVAILABLE FROM:-

Visual skills

Schools make demands upon pupils which can easily be taken for granted by both pupils and teachers. The teacher may assume that all mainstream pupils are able to hear adequately and see the printed word clearly on the page and white-board or blackboard. This may not be the case: some of the day-to-day routines pupils are asked to perform require skills and capabilities which they may not possess.

For example, when children are asked to copy from the board an extensive battery of skills is called upon:

(a) Enough attention to be able to focus on the board

(b) Adequate eyesight

(c) Ability to remember and find their place on the board

(d) Enough skill in handwriting to do write legibly

(e) Ability to keep the copied word in the mind for long enough to get in on paper accurately (visual memory)

(f) Knowledge that the words go from left to right across the board and from top to bottom

(g) Knowledge that the words go from left to right across the page and from top to bottom

On reflection, this apparently simple task is more complex than may be at first anticipated. Knowing the types of difficulty which dyslexic children have with short-term memory and sequencing skills, it is not surprising that they may find copying a demanding task.

Irlen syndrome

Some dyslexic children may not be able to see print clearly. A psychologist called Helen Irlen (see Booklist) claims that a particular group of children do not do so. She believes that they are experiencing a perceptual difficulty which she calls *'Scotopic Sensitivity Syndrome'* (SSS), also known as *'Irlen Syndrome'*. This syndrome has strong links with dyslexia. Many dyslexic children have difficulties with visual perception similar to those involved with the syndrome.

Children who experience the Irlen Syndrome appear to perceive some forms of writing in a distorted way. This is best explained in terms of their having an unusual sensitivity to certain wavelengths of light. This effect seems to be most pronounced with the colour contrast and glare of black print on shiny white paper under fluorescent light. This often describes the conditions under which children read in school. In class they will often find themselves sitting under a bright fluorescent light, reading a textbook which has bold black print on white paper or a whiteboard on which the teacher has written in black ink. Children describe the distorting effect this has in different ways, but almost all affected children speak of words appearing to move on the page, of them not keeping still, of them 'shivering', so that they are hard to read. Explaining this distortion is a task for optometrists (experts in vision), but the glare of the bright white light on the bright white page overloads the eye to the extent that it cannot efficiently process the information it sees.

Whatever the cause of the syndrome, the main ways of overcoming it are simple. They involve filtering out those parts of the light spectrum which are causing the distortion. This is achieved by the use of either coloured overlays placed over the text or by tinted filters set in spectacle frames. The correct shade of overlay is selected with children in an assessment conducted by trained screeners. Most LEAs employ some teachers or educational psychologists who can conduct this screen. If in doubt, the SENCO (see Glossary) at the school should know how to arrange an assessment or to be able to find out if not.

Overlays are inexpensive and can be very effective. Filters set in frames are very expensive and require a more skilled level of assessment. They are selected to suit individual requirements through an intensive one-to-one consultation with trained people called 'Diagnosticians'. The filters are made to specific requirements in California but adapted spectacles currently appear not to be available on prescription. Parents who wish to buy them for their children will almost always have to do so from their own pockets.

The jury is out on Irlen Syndrome. It is not a universally recognised medical condition. Our experience is that for some children overlays or tinted lenses seem to be very effective, but for others they do not work and can raise hopes unnecessarily high. A similar alternative is available in Britain called the 'Intuitive Colorimeter'. There is documentary evidence from children and adults who have benefited from using filters or overlays for reading. Their views cannot be ignored or dismissed, but should be handled with caution. It does not work for all but we would recommend that dyslexic children should be screened for overlays as part of their general assessment. If there is any doubt, if children seem to have difficulty perceiving words accurately, they should be taken to the local optician for assessment. They may not need overlays, but they may, unknown to you, have the kind of subtle visual deficiency which would not be picked up by the school-based eye tests. Eye tests at opticians are free for school-age children and they can only be arranged by parents not schools.

Making Allowance for Children's Dyslexia in Tests and Examinations

Throughout this book, we have stressed that when dyslexic children are being assessed, they need to be enabled to show fairly what they know. By this we mean that dyslexic children often have problems in demonstrating their knowledge and skills on paper. Their frequent difficulties in spelling, the inability of some children to sequence thoughts and ideas in writing, the problems others have in writing quickly and legibly, may all prevent them from fully showing their true potential in a subject. It is important that these children are given the maximum opportunity to demonstrate their true ability. This will sometimes mean that they must be allowed to take tests under different circumstances to other children. This is not a concession to them. It simply gives them a fairer starting point for examinations.

At this point we would like to make a few observations on the use made of national assessment scores. The results of Key Stage National Tests and GCSE examinations are reported to parents. They are also used to draw up league tables, which parents are encouraged to use to make comparisons between schools. This necessity to report Key Stage test results can be disadvantageous to children with special educational needs. It can make some schools reluctant to admit children, because it may pull their results down. This is a natural, if unfortunate reaction. Parents should look beyond the bare bones of these results when deciding which school they would like their children to attend. At the time of writing, investigations are being made into establishing a fairer way for schools' effectiveness to be measured than these unqualified results. The idea is to measure not only where children end up in terms of national test results, but also where they were on entry. Take two examples:

School A: School A has 90% of its 11-year-olds achieving Level 4 in English. This looks a wonderful record, 10% above the present Government's target of 80% achieving this standard. However, when you look back 4 years, you find that when the children entered the school, at the age of seven, 90% of them had already achieved Level 3. This means that in 4 years, the average child had only improved by one level: not much progress in this time, when they had done so well before. You would have thought they would at least be at Level 5 by now.

School B: Now look at School B. On the face of it, this school's results are worse than those for School A. At the end of Key Stage 2 only 70% of its pupils achieved Level 4 in English, 10% below the Government's target. However, if you again look at the children's scores 4 years before, you will find that the average score then was only Level 1. This means that, on average, the children in this school improved by two levels in 4 years; double the progress made by children in School A.

Which school has been the most effective in promoting the development of its pupils' English skills? Which school would be best for your dyslexic child? The decision is not as straightforward as it may at first have seemed.

Just as it is imperative for a school's results to be seen in context, so it is vital for individual children with special educational needs to be given the opportunity to show fairly the progress they have made. That is what this section is about.

Making allowances in school's internal tests and examinations

In the UK, the need to make allowances for some children when they sit examinations or tests is now widely acknowledged. Many mainstream schools make special allowances for dyslexic children when they take their own internal written examinations. They will arrange, for instance, that papers are read to some children. Alternatively, they might ensure that markers of some papers make allowance for poor handwriting or weak spelling. The markers may agree to mark work for content alone.

There is no legal requirement for schools to do this. However desirable it may be, it is their decision to do so. However, if children have a statement of special educational need (see Chapter 9), then it is possible for their statements to specify special conditions which should apply when they take internal examinations. This would need to have been negotiated with the school first, by the LEA. Alternatively, if children are above Stage 1 on the Special Needs Register, then their Individual Education Plan (see Chapter 8) may also state any allowances to be made for internal testing. If parents wish these kinds of allowance to be made, then they would normally discuss them in the first instance with the school's Special Needs Coordinator, probably at the time of a regular review meeting.

End of Key Stage National Tests (England and Wales)

These tests are called 'National Curriculum Assessments'. Children take them in the final year of the first three **Key Stages**:

Key Stage	Year of Test
One	Two
Two	Six
Three	Nine

Children must take these tests in English, Science and Mathematics (Welsh instead of English at Key Stage 1 in Welsh medium schools; Welsh and English in these schools at Key Stages 2 and 3). The agencies responsible for designing and over-seeing these tests have made considerable efforts to make them as accessible as possible for children with special educational needs. They aim to achieve this in several ways.

For Key Stage 2 tests only, if a teacher judges that children will not achieve higher on the tests than a Level 1 or 2, then they can be given alternative tasks as the basis of their assessments. These tasks allow children to demonstrate their knowledge in more practical ways. 'Task'-based results have equal status with ordinary test results. These arrangements are reviewed annually.

The main way in which allowance is made for individual needs, however, is that schools can make 'Special Arrangements' for some children. The idea of these arrangements is to allow children to more easily demonstrate their knowledge or skills, without making the test itself easier. Special arrangements must not provide an unfair advantage. Schools must ensure that any support given does not alter the nature of the test question and that the answer given is the pupil's own. This means that while teachers may be able to read questions to them, they cannot interpret the questions for the child. It means that while they may arrange to write a child's answers for him or her, they cannot use any words but those of the child. Rules and guidance for the kinds of arrangement which can be made, vary each year. The purpose of making special arrangements is to ensure that as many pupils as possible have access to the test, know what the assessment requires of them and have a suitable means of demonstrating their attainment. The tests themselves will be marked on an equal basis. The next box illustrates arrangements which a school can make at Key Stages 2 and 3, without external permission. It is hard to see how much more flexible and accommodating the test agencies could be for these children.

Special arrangements, which may be useful for dyslexic children, and which do not need external permission. Permission may be given by the headteacher.

- Read the papers to the child (or a taped version can be made)

- Write a child's answers (also known as 'amanuensis')

- Use real objects instead of pictures and diagrams for Science

- Separate the test into sections: to give children rest breaks

- Use of coloured overlays for visual clarity

- Enhancement of diagrams (i.e. to help children with spatial difficulties)

- Use of mechanical and technological aids (e.g. word-processors — not for handwriting; spellcheckers — not for English/Welsh spelling/writing)

- Provide a transcript: if the child's handwriting is illegible

- Taking the test in a separate room

However, schools must apply for external permission for the following arrangements:

- Open a paper early (to make special preparations for the child to take the test)

- Allow the child to have extra time to complete the test (up to 25% extra)

A named LEA officer is designated to have responsibility for vetting such requests. Schools use a special form to apply to the LEA for permission. On this form they have to say what kind of special arrangement is being sought, and provide evidence for the request. Usually this evidence would be in the form of the child's Individual Education Plan. LEA officers must decide whether they agree with the request. If they do agree, then they sign the form and return it to the school, with a covering letter granting permission. The Test Agencies keep a careful eye on the use of special arrangements. They may visit a school at any time during the test period, to check that they are being used fairly.

It should be stressed that the statementing procedure has no bearing on special arrangements for Key Stage National Tests. Some children with a statement will not be granted permission to have special arrangements made for them. Other children without statements will be granted them. It is a matter for the school to identify those children for whom it believes require special arrangements to be made. However, it would be unusual for special arrangements to be granted by the LEA for a child who was not at Stage 3 or above on the Special Educational Needs Register.

Dispensation for the General Certificate of Secondary Education Examinations

In England and Wales, at the age of 16, nearly all children will take national examinations called the General Certificate of Secondary Education (GCSE). If they remain in school after the age of 16, most children will take Advanced Level examinations at the age of 18. For both sets of examination, schools can apply for 'dispensation' for some children with special educational needs. To do so they have to follow this process:

Procedure for applying for GCSE/'A' level dispensation

(1) School decides that the severity of a particular child's special educational needs indicate that dispensations may be necessary.

(2) The school arranges for the child to be assessed by an educational psychologist, with dispensation in mind. At the time of writing it seems likely that specially

trained teachers will also be allowed to make these assessments. Check with your school's examination officer.

(3) The psychologist assesses the child and determines whether or not dispensation is appropriate.

(4) The psychologist formally reports back to school in writing on the child's need for dispensation.

(5) If the psychologist has agreed, then the school will apply for dispensation to the Examination Board concerned, using the psychologist's report as evidence.

(6) Each Examination Board has its own criteria for determining if dispensation is necessary. They will check the school's request and the psychologist's report against these criteria. If the child's needs meets the criteria, then dispensation will be formally granted in writing to the school.

As with Key Stage National Tests, the statementing procedure plays no part in this decision-making. Children do not need a statement to be granted dispensation for GCSE or 'A' Level examinations. The form of dispensation to be sought for a particular child would normally be discussed by the psychologist, parents and special needs coordinator. The kinds of dispensation allowed vary from Examination Board to Examination Board. **Typical kinds of dispensation** are:

- Extra time at the beginning of the examination

- Extra time at the end of an examination

- Supervised rest breaks

- Paper read to candidate (or taped recording of paper)

- Answers written down by a scribe, usually a teacher (Amanuensis)

- Dictation of answers on to tape

- Use of a word-processor to write answers

- Allowance can be made for spelling, punctuation and grammar: but paper may be endorsed to this effect

Examination Boards are strict about granting dispensations. They are, correctly, determined to maintain the integrity of their assessments. They only grant dispensations if they are essential for the children, in order that they may show what they know. The Boards will only allow dispensations which do not make the examination itself easier. Some dispensations — e.g. allowance for spelling — do not, for obvious reasons, apply to English or Welsh Language examinations.

The best time to consider seeking dispensations for children is during Year 9 before children begin their GCSE courses. This is for two reasons. Firstly, educational psychologists almost always have huge demands on their time. They need to be given as much forewarning as possible that they need to make an assessment on a child. Secondly, many GCSE courses are modular. This means that they are taught in a sequence of modules, each of which is tested as the child completes it. Therefore, children may be taking GCSE examinations during Year 10, not just at the end of Year 11. If they are entitled to dispensation, then this entitlement may also apply to modular course examinations. The psychologist will, in these circumstances, need to make his or her assessment early enough for the school to apply to the Board, and receive permission, before the modular test is taken. Schools and parents need to be fully aware of children's rights in this area of dispensation and special arrangements. These allowances are a right, an entitlement, not a privilege. The examinations are not being made easier. All that is happening is that the child with special educational needs is being offered a playing field which is as level as it can be, when compared to that made available for other children.

Some children, especially older pupils, may not accept the special arrangements or dispensations which have been made for them. For instance they may refuse to have papers read to them, because it makes them stand out. Although they have been granted extra time, they may leave the examination room at the same time as the others, for the same reason. There is no easy answer to this. Probably it is best to allow each child to decide for him or herself. Quite often it is enough for the child to know that they can take extra time, if it is needed. This knowledge can be reassurance enough, even if ultimately they find that they do not actually need to use it.

Understanding Assessment Reports Written by External Specialists

At some time, as a teacher or parent of a dyslexic child, you are likely to receive a detailed assessment report from a specialist in the field, usually someone not attached to the child's school. This person might be a state-employed educational psychologist or learning support teacher. It might be a private psychologist or teacher. Our advice to parents is to use the services of their local authority first. You have paid for it in your taxes and it is an entitlement for your child. In the UK, if an assessment by an educational psychologist is necessary, then all children who live in a local authority area are entitled to it free. This applies to children in private schools. Only when you have had such an assessment done and are unhappy with it should you need to look elsewhere. This is rarely needed. The great majority of LEA-employed educational psychologists are highly trained and experienced former teachers who will give parents and schools expert advice which is independent of the LEA. Specialist learning support teachers attached to the LEA are equally valuable sources of information and guidance.

Psychologists and teachers will tend to assess children from different perspectives. The former will concentrate on explaining why the child has a difficulty and precisely defining it. The latter will usually emphasise the specific teaching programmes which are needed in more detail. A combination of both is the ideal. Within England and Wales (see the next chapter), external assessment reports are frequently written for children at Stage 3 of the Code of Practice (these reports will be written by either an educational psychologist or a specialist teacher or both. They are always written for children being assessed for statutory assessment (Appendix F of the statementing process must be written by an educational psychologist).

At one time, many of these reports were often quite difficult for parents and teachers to understand. They were full of jargon and complex technical language which seemed to be designed to impress or confuse, rather than enlighten the reader. Most report writers now make a conscious attempt to present their findings in plain English and to explain the technical terms they use. In case they do not, we will end this chapter with our guide to assessment reports. In this we have identified the most common jargon used in them and attempted to explain them in straightforward language:

Understanding the terms used in reports

Term used	*What it means*
Receptive language	Children's ability to understand what is said to them.
Expressive language	Their ability to communicate their thoughts and feelings in speech.
Fine motor skills	Small movements of the body, typically finger and hand movements, like drawing or tying laces.
Gross motor skills	Large movements of the limbs and body, like running, hopping, throwing and catching.
Hand–eye Coordination	How well the brain gets the hand to do what the eye is telling it to do! Comments on this usually concerns skills like tracing and writing.
Short-term memory	How well information is held in children's working memory.
Short-term visual memory	Ability to remember information which has been seen.
Short-term auditory memory	Ability to remember information which has been heard.
Visual perception	How accurately children see information. This usually refers to their ability to correctly see the shapes made by words, letters and numbers.
Auditory perception	How accurately children hear information. This usually refers to their ability to correctly hear the sounds made by words, letters and numbers.

Term used	What it means
Cognitive ability	This refers to children's ability to think and reason.
Quotient	A quotient is a useful way of showing children's scores on a test compared to the average which would be expected if all children were tested on it. Average scores usually lie between 89–111 with a mean of 100.
IQ	This stands for Intelligence Quotient. IQ tests are controversial. Some psychologists will not use them. They say they lack validity. One thing seems certain: children who do well in IQ tests tend to do well in exams, when right answers are required for closed questions. They are good predictors of how well children will perform in school. They are measures of children's potential. The importance for dyslexic children, therefore, can be that their IQ test will show that in comparison to their school potential measured by the IQ test they are under-performing. IQ scores are not fixed. Appropriate teaching can significantly raise them.
The British Ability Scales or BAS	This is the title of the IQ test used most frequently by British Educational Psychologists. It gives three self-explanatory summary scores: Visual IQ, Verbal IQ and a general IQ. Watch out for the difference between the visual and verbal score. A large discrepancy is a significant indication that children have a dyslexic type difficulty.
The Weschler Intelligence Scale for Children (WISC)	Another very commonly used IQ test. It should be an Anglicised version of the original American test.
ACID profile (ACID = Arithmetic, Coding, Information and Digit Span)	The report may say that the ACID profile is present. This refers to four sub-tests of the WISC Test which are strong indicators of a dyslexic type problem. If children have been given the WISC test look out for their ACID scores. The sub-tests are: Arithmetic, Coding, Information and Digit Span. Saying children have an ACID profile means that the tester believes their low scores on these tests is accompanied by higher scores in other sub-tests, thus strongly suggesting the presence of dyslexia.

The next items deal with the BAS sub-tests which are most frequently used to assess children who may be dyslexic.

Speed of information-processing	How quickly problems can be solved. Children have to solve a sequence of number problems against the clock. They get progressively harder.
Matrices	This test closely resembles the lay-person's idea of an IQ test. They are a test of non-verbal reasoning ability or the ability to reason without words. Typically children are shown a pattern of shapes and have to work out the next one in the sequence.

Term used	What it means
Similarities	This is a measure of verbal reasoning or reasoning with words. Children are given two words and then asked to say how they are similar.
Block design	This is a test of visual spatial ability. It measures children's ability to see shapes in relation to each other. Children are given a number of differently patterned cubes. A picture of a pattern which can be made with the cubes is shown to them. They have to reproduce it against the clock.
Copying	Exactly as it sounds: it measures children's skill in seeing shapes and accurately reproducing them. Children are shown a shape and then asked to copy it.
Immediate visual recall	This is a test of short-term memory. Children are shown a card on which are 20 simple pictures. They have 2 minutes to try and remember as many pictures as possible. Then the card is turned over and they have to recall them.
Delayed visual recall	Twenty minutes later they are asked to recall them again.
Recall of designs	This test measures short-term memory and motor skills. Children are shown a picture of a shape for five seconds. Then the picture is withdrawn and they have to draw it from memory.
Recall of digits	This assesses short-term auditory memory. The tester says a sequence of numbers slowly. Children then have to repeat the numbers in the correct sequence. The sequences get longer.
Basic number skills	This mainly tests arithmetic skills. It does not assess the whole of mathematics. It is quite possible for children to perform badly on this test but be much more able in other areas of maths — just as some children's spelling is poor but their creative writing is excellent. This test will give a number age score which can be compared to the general IQ score to see whether they are is performing at their potential.
Word definitions	This is a measure of vocabulary and of children's ability to understand words and express that understanding.
Word reading	This tests children's ability to read single words in isolation. As with mathematics, some dyslexic children will score better on other areas of reading. This test can give a reading age score which, like the number test, can be compared to the general IQ score to see if they are performing at their potential.
Spiky profile	This term is used when children's performance on the different sub-tests is not even. Typically, dyslexic children will score well on tests like 'similarities' or 'matrices', but poorly on recall of digits or visual recall. This will give an uneven or spiky profile which is often taken to indicate that children have a dyslexic type difficulty. Some psychologists helpfully show the test scores in a series of bar graphs. This quickly shows if there is a spiky profile.

Term used	What it means

Other terms which may be used

Reading accuracy age	This is a measure of how well children read the precise text in front of them. Dyslexic children will often not perform so well in this aspect of reading.
Reading comprehension age	This measures how well children have understood the meaning of the text. Fortunately, dyslexic children will tend to do better in this skill which is, after all, what we read for.
Reading fluency age	Despite its name this is not a measure of how smoothly and naturally children read. It actually measures how fast they read. Watch out for a high fluency age and a low accuracy or comprehension age. This will indicate they are rushing to complete the task without thinking of the real purpose of reading. Such children will need to be taught and encouraged to become more reflective and attentive readers.

Summary of Chapter 7

This chapter:

- described the kinds of skill which children need in nearly all subjects across the curriculum including perception, memory and recall;

- looked further at using mind-maps and mnemonics, to help children plan and structure their learning;

- showed how chunking information, and using rhyme and rhythm, can help children learn;

- discussed how children can improve their exam revision technique;

- showed the effects of being dyslexic on children's performance in different subjects across the curriculum;

- described how dyslexic children can organise themselves better in school;

- covered the concept of Irlen Syndrome;

- described the allowances which can be made for dyslexic children when they take national tests;

- provided a guide to understanding the terms used in some experts' reports on children.

Chapter 8

The Code of Practice on the Identification and Assessment of Special Educational Needs

This chapter concentrates on responsibilities which schools and parents have towards children with special needs, including dyslexic children. It begins with the principles upon which the Code is built and then describes the role of the school based Special Needs Coordinator and the contents of the Special Needs Policy which every school must have. It finishes with a detailed description of the Code's first three assessment stages. Although it is primarily concerned with the UK system, most countries maintain similar procedures for the identification and assessment of children with special educational needs. It bears many similarities to the system used in many North American States.

Background

The Code of Practice (COP) is contained within the UK's 1996 Education Act. It lays down recommendations and ground-rules for education authorities, schools, parents and other agencies in their work with children with special educational needs. The **scope of the code of practice** is as follows.

- **Identification**   Finding out that the child has a difficulty.

- **Assessment**   Establishing in detail the nature of the difficulty.

- **Provision**   Providing what the child needs to overcome the difficulty.

- **Review**   Monitoring the provision to make sure the difficulty is being overcome.

It does not cover non-maintained schools or nurseries, although these may voluntarily adopt the same system. Although at one point it does make specific reference to dyslexic pupils, the Code is mainly concerned with guidelines which are common to all children with special needs, including dyslexics. Good practice for one is seen as good practice for all children.

Dyslexic children are not, in this respect, different from all other children with special educational needs. They require many of the same services: early accurate identification of children's difficulties should lead to specific programmes which will assist them to achieve their full potential in school.

Most of the Code of Practice is not compulsory. Where it is compulsory, we will make this clear. However, schools, education authorities and other agencies must *'have regard'* to it. It cannot be ignored. Schools must plan their provision in its light. What this actually means in practice is something like the following:

> Schools need not follow the Code in its every detail. However, their policy and provision for special needs should reflect what is in the Code. In practice schools must have something in place which is at least as effective as the Code.

So although the Code does not say you must do it this way, its writers are saying something like this:

> We know schools are doing their best to meet the needs of all their pupils. However, there is a great variation between the way different schools provide for special needs and we believe there should be more consistency of approach. Therefore, we have designed a blueprint for schools to refer to, to measure their practice against. Schools should be aware of the Code's guidelines and make sure that its policy and practice are in line with them.

The Main Features of the Code of Practice

The following table outlines the main provisions of the Code.

Guideline or Regulation	Main Feature
Several key principles are identified. These are intended to underpin good practice in identifying and meeting children's needs.	Practices and procedures essential to achieving these principles are listed.
Every school must have a special needs policy.	It must be available to parents.
Every school should have a Special Needs Co-ordinator (SENCO).	Responsible for the day-to-day running of the policy.
Every school should have a designated Special Needs Governor.	Responsible to the Governing Body for oversight of the running of the policy.
There should be a staged approach to assessing and monitoring a child's special needs.	Five stages are recommended.
All agencies involved with children with special needs should work closely and cooperatively together to assess their needs and make provision which meets them.	The Code has guidelines and instructions for Child Health Services and Social Service Departments.
Regulations are laid down for the procedure called Statutory Assessment which may lead to a child having a statement made out for him or her.	This procedure is commonly called 'statementing'. The Code says that it should be fairer and quicker with more detailed outcomes for each child. Parents' rights of appeal are strengthened.

The Principles, Practice and Procedure Which Underpin the Code

The COP is based on several important principles which you need to know. In the chart below we have given a typical example of how each principle might apply to dyslexic children:

EARLY IDENTIFICATION AND ASSESSMENT IS ESSENTIAL	**IDENTIFIED NEEDS MUST BE ADDRESSED**	**CHILDREN WITH SPECIAL NEEDS ARE ENTITLED TO A BROAD AND BALANCED CURRICULUM**
Dyslexic children can be identified as early as five years old and should be identified by the time they are seven.	Dyslexic children often need specific approaches such as multi-sensory teaching.	This is very true of dyslexic pupils who are intellectually able to follow the whole curriculum.

MINOR DIFFICULTIES NEED MINOR PROVISION, MAJOR DIFFICULTIES NEED MAJOR PROVISION	**THE KNOWLEDGE, VIEWS AND EXPERIENCE OF PARENTS ARE VITAL**
The severity of a child's difficulty is crucial. Some children may need little more than a little bit of extra help, others may need regular small group teaching with a specialist teacher. It is important that the severity of children's difficulties are accurately established.	Most schools welcome parents' views and seek to fully involve them in their work with the child. Some are less keen. Do not be put off by being made to feel anxious, fussy or protective.

MOST CHILDREN WILL HAVE THEIR NEEDS MET IN THEIR LOCAL MAINSTREAM SCHOOL WITHOUT THE NEED FOR STATUTORY ASSESSMENT	**STATUTORY ASSESSMENT SHOULD BE EFFICIENT, CLEAR AND THOROUGH**	**THINGS WORK BEST WHEN EVERYONE, INVOLVED INCLUDING THE CHILD, WORK TOGETHER IN PARTNERSHIP**
As long they are given the correct help there, dyslexic children belong in mainstream schools. It is not in their best interests to attend special schools.	It is essential that the assessment states that the child has specific learning difficulties, identifies what those difficulties are and states the provision necessary to help the child overcome them.	This is obviously true but it easy to overlook the child when making decisions about him or her. The general rules are: listen to them, help them express their point of view and act on it.

The Special Educational Needs Policy

The Code states that every school must have a special educational needs (SEN) policy. In the annual report to parents there must be a section stating how the SEN policy has been carried out. The school prospectus must also have a summary of the policy. All of this is compulsory. The Code does not say exactly what should be in the policy, but it lists a number of headings which it should address. These are shown in the table.

This requirement for schools to have an SEN Policy is a vital new development and potentially a rich source of information for parents and teachers. Correctly written, a school's SEN policy should give a clear insight into the value the school places on its pupils with SEN and how well organised it is to make appropriate provision for them. It is sometimes interesting to compare the school's statement of principle towards children with special needs with the actual proportion of its budget which it is prepared to allocate to them. Fine words do not butter parsnips. However, do not judge too quickly. A school which does not spend as much funding as you might expect on, for instance, employing a special needs teacher, may be so superbly organised, have so excellent a curriculum and have such small classes, that it does not need a special needs teacher so often.

SEN policies can become the firm foundation of every school's SEN provision or yet another piece of paper filling the Headteacher's filing cabinet. The most central factors in their success are the school's commitment to implement them and parents' insistence on their implementation.

The contents of the school's SEN policy

General area	Specific information required	Comment
(A) Basic information about the school's SEN provision	Objectives and principles	You should be able to work out if the school values its pupils with special needs in this section.
	The Special Needs Coordinator should be identified	This person could well be your main contact in the school.
	Arrangements for coordinating SEN Provision	E.g. how much time has the Coordinator got to perform his or her duties?
	Admission arrangements for pupils with SEN	The policy should make it clear that the school would not prevent children being admitted simply because they have special needs.
	Details of SEN specialisms which the school caters or facilities for pupils with SEN which it may house	e.g. the school may have extra resources for specific kinds of special need, including dyslexia.

General area	Specific information required	Comment
(B) How children's needs are identified, assessed and met	How resources are allocated to and among pupils with SEN	The policy should state how much the school is given by the LEA or Funding Council for children with special needs, how much if any, it adds to that sum and how it is spent.
	How needs are identified and reviewed	Each school should have a clearly stated process which shows how children's difficulties are identified and monitored.
	How pupils with SEN have access to a broad and balanced curriculum	A broad and balanced curriculum is compulsory for all children.
	How well pupils with SEN integrate	This is particularly important for children in a special school or in a 'unit' attached to an ordinary school.
	How SEN provision is evaluated	This is vital. The Governing Body have a duty to see that provision is appropriate to children's needs.
	How parents may complain about the provision made for SEN	The policy should describe a clear process.
(C) Information about staffing policies and outside agencies	Arrangements for in-service training	The policy should state how teachers will be trained, individually or as a whole, to teach children with special needs.
	Use of outside agencies	Effective liaison with outside agencies is vital. A good policy will list the key contact people for each agency. Look out especially for the name of the educational psychologist probably assigned to the school.
	Role of parents of children with SEN	Hopefully the policy will acknowledge the vital role which parents have and how the school intends to make it possible for parents to play this role.
	Links with other schools	Look especially for links with the next school in line — infant to junior, junior to secondary, secondary to further education college.
	Links with health and social services	Minimum information is the names of the school nurse and doctor, the number of the local social service department. The better policy will state how good liaison with these agencies is fostered and maintained.

The Special Educational Needs Coordinator (SENCO)

The Code of Practice states that every school should have a Special Educational Needs Coordinator or SENCO. As the name suggests, this teacher has the main responsibility for the day-to-day implementation of the school's special needs policy. The Governors and the Headteacher make the policy. The SENCO makes the policy happen. (In many schools, the Headteacher is also the SENCO.) The main duties of the SENCO are given in the diagram below.

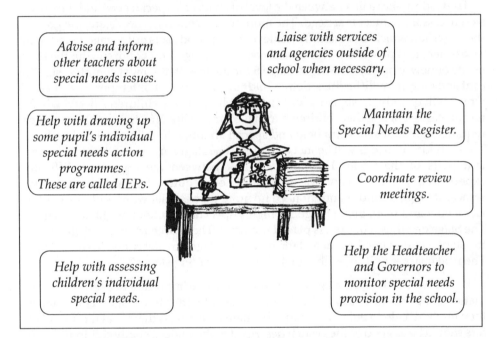

Advise and inform other teachers about special needs issues.

Liaise with services and agencies outside of school when necessary.

Help with drawing up some pupil's individual special needs action programmes. These are called IEPs.

Maintain the Special Needs Register.

Coordinate review meetings.

Help with assessing children's individual special needs.

Help the Headteacher and Governors to monitor special needs provision in the school.

It is a busy job. Many SENCOs, especially those in primary schools, are full-time class or subject teachers. They often do not have the time to coordinate as effectively as they would like. The Government viewed the introduction of the Code as being 'cost neutral': in other words they did not believe it would cost more money to implement. Therefore, it did not allocate extra resources to help schools deliver the Code procedures. Experience has shown this to have been rather unrealistic. Many schools simply do not have the money to fund it properly.

Parents are not helpless in this. Each year the school's budget must be presented to them by the Governors at the Annual General Meeting. Parents of children with SEN should attend this meeting. They should look at the printed budget summary and note how much is allocated to special needs. If they think it is insufficient, they should say so at the meeting. If the Governors can show they had no alternative because of the restrictions imposed by the overall budget, parents should raise this with their local councillor or MP, or with the LEA or the Funding Council. Remember support for pupils with special needs is a partnership between home and school. The role of parents in securing adequate resources for SEN in their children's school can be vital.

The Five Stages of Assessment for Children with Special Needs

The Code makes a link between the level of children's special need and the provision necessary to meet that need. The more severe children's needs are, the greater the provision which is needed. To achieve this the Code sets out a staged model for assessment and provision. This model goes from Stage 1 for children with the least needs or newly detected needs to Stage 5 for those with the most complex, significant and long-term difficulties. Some children have a minor or temporary difficulty which will quickly disappear given the right help. These children's needs will be met at Stages 1 or 2. Other children may have a major life-affecting condition which requires a great deal of extra help and special attention for all their time in school. These children's needs will be met at Stage 5. The stages are one of the most important parts of the Code. They make a link between the degree of difficulty experienced by children and the amount of help required to overcome it. For instance, at Stage 1 children might need no more than a quiet word with the teacher alone now and then, but at Stage 5 a highly specialised school might be essential. The Stage on which children is placed is crucial. The flowchart on p.179 illustrates the stages. Following this, each of the first three stages are described in some detail. The next chapter will cover the final two 'Statementing stages'.

Before we describe the stages, you will need some important background information about them. Firstly, schools do not need to offer five stages. For instance, they might decide to only offer four. The main principle is that what the school offers should be as good as the system described in the Code. Usually children should go through one stage before they can be considered for the next. However, where it is obviously necessary, children can be moved more quickly or 'fast-tracked' through the stages. Typical examples of fast-tracked pupils are those whose education has been severely affected by injury in a road traffic accident, or children who suddenly acquire a major hearing or vision loss, or children for whom some trauma has caused them to have sudden and severe behavioural problems. Children do not need to automatically go through the stages from one to five. Most will go no further than Stage 2. Each stage will now be described in detail.

Outline of the first three stages of assessment and provision

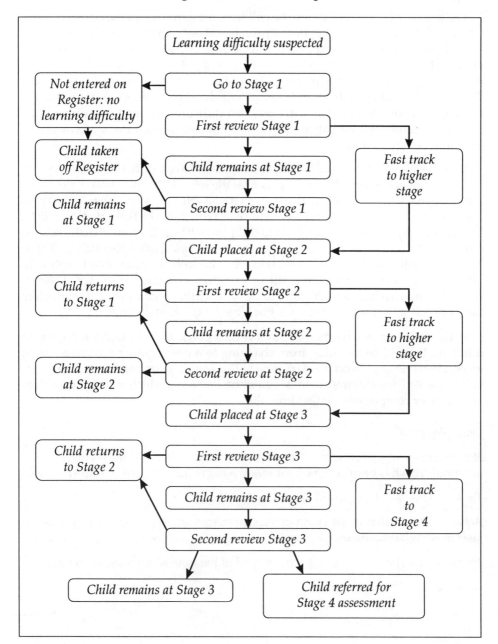

Stage 1

The key people at this stage are the children, the parents and the class or subject teachers. What will usually happen at primary school is that the teacher or the parent will notice that children appear to have a difficulty with some aspect of school. They will then consult with each other. This need not be on a formal basis: a brief note might go home or the parent might ask to see the teacher after school one day. The teacher would also inform and consult with the SENCO. At secondary school, it is more likely that the teacher will observe a difficulty and will consult with the SENCO, informing parents about the desired outcome of their discussion and asking for their views on this.

If it is decided that the children have or appear to have a difficulty, then they will be entered on the Special Needs Register for the school. Parents should always be informed that this has happened. In consultation with the parents an informal plan of action will be decided on and recorded. This record will be brief, its aims will be limited and any extra attention given to children will be minor and usually offered only by the 'ordinary' teacher and/or parent. Some typical examples of Stage 1 aims and actions will now follow. The idea is to solve the problem quickly and easily or to establish that there is a significant difficulty which needs a higher level of 'differentiation'. If children have learning difficulties you will hear the word 'differentiation' rather frequently. It is a very simple, but a very important concept:

Differentiation is what is done to a child's curriculum to make it special or different. It could be anything from changing to a new reading scheme to being given a behaviour contract, to extra time with a learning support teacher, to toilets being adapted for children with a disability: anything which will help children overcome or compensate for the difficulty.

Example: John

Nature of concern: John is four. He screams and cries when Mum tries to leave him in school. This has been going on for many weeks with no signs of improvement.

Target: John will leave his Mum without crying.

Action: Mum will stay with John in class for an ever shorter time each day as he adjusts to being without her.

Monitoring: The teacher will keep a record of the time Mum stays each day.

Review date: Six weeks time.

Example: Tracey

Nature of concern: Tracey is seven and is beginning to fall behind her classmates in spelling. It is not a major problem. Typically she keeps on spelling some awkward little words wrong. The trouble is they are very common words like 'was', 'were', 'to' and 'the'.

Target: Tracey will be able to spell accurately, every time, the 20 words she most commonly misspells.

Action: Tracey will practice the words in groups of five at home using a special method called 'Look–Picture–Cover–Write–Check'. The teacher will give her a weekly test on the words.

Monitoring: The weekly test.

Review date: End of term.

Example: Penny

Nature of concern: Penny is 13 and beginning to drift away from school. She is late nearly every day and she is frequently absent. She is bright and not a behaviour problem in other ways, at home or school.

Target: To be on time for school on 90% of possible half days.

Action: Her form tutor will explain why everyone is worried about her. Her parents have agreed to do the same. She will keep a punctuality chart. Every week she is punctual for nine out of ten sessions she will be given a simple reward by her parents. (Allowed out for an extra hour on Saturday night.)

Monitoring: The punctuality chart.

Review date: Six weeks time.

Reviewing progress at Stage 1

When deciding on the action plan, a date to review its success must be set. A reasonable time at this stage is from 6 weeks to 3 months — enough to give the plan a chance to work without the danger of leaving it so long it gets significantly worse. The review sees how close children have got to the target. Usually the review would simply consist of the class-teacher talking to parents perhaps with the SENCO and the child present. It can have several outcomes:

Possible outcomes of Stage 1 reviews

Conclusion of review	Possible outcome
The difficulty is resolved. Children have completely overcome the problem.	Note it in their record and monitor progress.
The difficulty seems to be resolved but it is not certain.	Stop the action plan and review progress in three months time.
Children have made some progress but have not overcome the difficulty.	Keep the plan running for a further three months and see how they are then doing.
The difficulty is significantly greater. There is now concern that without urgent intervention from a specialist external to the school a major difficulty will develop.	Consider a move to Stage 3 immediately.
The difficulty is now greater. There is concern about children's ability to overcome the problem at Stage 1.	Consider a move to Stage 2 immediately.
Children have not responded to the plan. The difficulty is not significantly worse but it hasn't changed either.	Adapt the plan, try a new strategy and review in three months.

Stage 2

The key people at this stage are the child, the parents, the class or subject teachers and the SENCO. The major difference between Stages 1 and 2 is that, at this stage, an Individual Educational Plan (IEP) should be drawn up for the children. This will be more formal and more detailed than the kind of plan used at Stage 1. It will be written down as a simple blueprint for the teachers to follow. At Stage 2, the SENCO has a more important role. This is one of responsibility for ensuring that the IEP is drawn up and implemented. The SENCO may not actually write it but should make sure it is appropriate to the child's needs. In many schools, placement at Stage 2 will mean that a teacher with responsibility for teaching special needs in the school will be assigned to the child.

The SENCO is also responsible for ensuring the IEP is implemented and the child's progress on it reviewed. The review period will vary according to the child. Usually a maximum of 6 and a minimum of 3 months will be set for the next review. However, some children may remain at Stage 2 for several years. This is nothing to worry about. It should mean that they have a difficulty which is at least being contained by the action the school is taking to meet it. If the child is making proper progress at this stage, then the review period can be gradually increased up to a maximum of 12 months.

What is an Individual Education Plan (IEP)

The IEP is a blueprint. It should set out to where you want children to travel, how they are to travel and how you will know when they have arrived. A **typical Stage 2 individual education plan** should contain the following:

- a brief description of the child's learning difficulties;
- the provision to be made to meet those difficulties;
- targets to be aimed at;
- staff involved;
- when the programme is to be carried out;
- specific programmes/equipment;
- the role of parents in supporting the IEP;
- any pastoral care or medical requirements;
- how success in achieving targets is to be gauged.

Parents are entitled to know what is in their child's IEP and to have a copy of it. It is possible that some schools will charge for a photocopy of the IEP. An example of a typical Stage 2 IEP is given on the opposite page.

Setting targets

The setting of specific targets for children is the key to the whole process. To set a target, the school must decide the kind of progress they expect children to make and specify it. This will mean that the teachers have something to measure the effectiveness of the IEP against. The target should state the skills, concepts or knowledge which children are expected to learn and state criteria whose achievement will indicate the target has been reached. If we took spelling as an example of this process, then a possible target might be:

To improve his spelling.

But this is too vague and woolly. It needs to be more precise. Improve spelling of what? We need to try again and be clearer about exactly what we want to be achieved.

To be able to spell simple three letter words.

This does not tell us much more. We would want it to be more precise. We would want to know what kind of three letter words. A better target might be:

STAGE TWO

I.E.P

Exemplar

Individual Education Plan

Name

Stephen Alan Richards

Age

| 9 | Years | 3 | Months |

Class / Form	N.C. Yr	SEN Stage	I.E.P. Date	Next Review Date
Mrs Jones	5	2	29 Sep, 96	Feb 97

Reading Age	6.9
Spelling Age	6.7
Numeracy Age	8.9

Tel 014523765

Are parents able / willing to help support at home
- ● Yes
- O No

I.E.P. Monitoring by:
- ☐ Headteacher
- ☒ SENCO
- ☒ Class teacher
- ☐ Subject teacher
- ☐ Pastoral Head
- ☒ Parent
- ☐ External Agencies
- ☐ Key Worker

Medical/Pastoral requirements

None

Pen portrait of the pupil

Alan is a lively orally bright child who is struggling with acquiring a level of literacy appropriate to his ability in other areas. His parents are very supportive and very willing to hep at home.   He has just been placed on stage two and will receive two half hour sessions from the school's learning support teacher to help offer the programmes identified below.

TARGET: It is intended that by the next review adequate progress will enable the pupil to :-	PROVISION: The following provision will normally be made available :-	TARGET ACHIEVED: with date and/or comment :-
read with understanding	A home-school reading programme based on the Reading 360 books and reinforced by extra reading at school.	
when reading to use phonic knowledge of :	Regular sessions with learning support teacher for appropriate phonic programes.	
recognise on sight	A programme to develop ability to recognise the McNally Murray words based on simple memory games.	
spell words which can be read on sight	A programme based on the look-visualise -cover-visualise- write-check method	
recognise and use these simple spelling patterns: consonant and vowel digraphs.	A programme with the learning support teacher on recognising and using these spelling patterns:	

This review recommends that   Stephen   will remain at Stage Two

(with thanks to Roger Hayward and Malcolm Brockley of Denbighshire LEA for the design of this IEP)

To be able to spell regular 'c-v-c' words.

This is more precise. (By the way, 'c-v-c' words are made up of a consonant (c) a short vowel (v) and a another consonant (c): words like fat, hen, bit, top, cut. See the phonics section of Chapter 2.) But it does not give us a criteria for success. Will the child be expected to spell every c–v–c word accurately every time or half the time or most times? The target needs to be more specific here:

To be able to spell regular 'c-v-c' words nine times out of ten.

There is still something missing. We know what the child should be able to do, and how often s/he should be doing it. We do not know when or where it should be achieved. We all know children who get 20/20 every week in the spelling test after parents have helped them learn them at home, but who then spell those same words wrong in a story the next week. So the target needs to include when and where it should be achieved. In our example it might be as follows:

To be able to spell regular 'c-v-c' words nine times out of ten in his own unaided writing.

This is the kind of target we would recommend for an IEP at Stage 2. It is simple to write and its achievement is simple to assess. The criteria for success will vary from child to child. For some children, 90% accuracy would be unrealistic, for others 100% could be achievable.

A target should, wherever possible, be measurable. To show that children have achieved a target you must be able to see or hear it being achieved. This is where the criteria are so important. The next table lists examples of targets in a range of areas related to children with dyslexic difficulties. They are given as possibilities. Different schools and teachers will have different ways of working. But each one is 'seeable' or 'hearable' and therefore measurable. One caution for parents and teachers. Some things are easily measured but are not important and vice versa. The main principle which schools will aim at here is to make the important measurable not the measurable important.

Examples of typical IEP targets

Area	Target
Reading	Will be able to read Oxford Reading Tree Level 3 books with 90% accuracy.
Reading	Will be able to read the 32 most common English words as they occur in her reading with 90% accuracy.
Spelling	Will be able to spell her own name and address with no more than two mistakes.

Area	Target
Spelling	Will be able to write accurately 'c-v-c' words when they are said to him, eight times out of ten.
Writing	Will be able to identify 8/10 spelling mistakes in his free writing and attempt to correct them using a special dictionary.
Writing	Will always correctly use ascenders and descenders d, h, p and g in her free writing.
Mathematics	Will be able to say her five and six times tables by heart with no errors.
Mathematics	Will always write '3 and 5' the correct way round when working on calculations.
Memory	Will always check his daily equipment schedule at home before packing his school bag

Secondary schools may set targets which will apply to most or nearly all subjects. These are called cross-curricular targets. They are especially important at secondary school because of the large number of different subjects and teachers which children will encounter there each week. Here are some common examples of cross-curricular targets in secondary schools:

Area	Target
Presentation	Will always underline the title and date each piece of work.
Spelling	Will always spell 'there' and 'their' correctly.
Reading	Will ask for help when stuck on a word.
Behaviour	Will arrive at the lesson on time.

How many targets?

How many targets should be set? We would suggest that children's needs are prioritised with no more than two or three specific areas. To try for more than this would be unrealistic at Stage 2.

Reviewing progress at Stage 2

As with Stage 1, Stage 2 reviews should be held before a decision can be made to move children between stages. Exceptional circumstances can mean that children are moved sooner than this. The main focus of the review meetings should be to see how well children have progressed towards their targets. To save time and be more efficient, the school may well time a review to coincide with a routine parents' evening. **Some possible outcomes of Stage 2 review are:**

Conclusion of review	Possible outcome
The child's difficulties appear to have been overcome.	Return to Stage 1 and monitor progress
The child has made some progress but has not overcome the difficulty.	Continue with Stage 2
The child's difficulties are now comparatively greater. The school require specialist intervention in designing the IEP.	Move to Stage 3 and refer child to appropriate agency for assessment and advice.
The child's difficulties have increased to a level where the school believe his or her educational needs cannot be met without resources over and above those available in an ordinary school.	Referral of the child to an appropriate agency seeking advice on child's need for statutory assessment.

Stage 3

The key people at this stage are the children, the parents, the class or subject teachers, the SENCO and an outside agency called in to give specialist advice. The major difference between Stage 3 and Stage 2 is that the former involves an outside specialist in helping the school design and monitor the IEP. There are several different kinds of specialist who might become involved at Stage 3. Do not be alarmed by the term 'specialist'. For dyslexic pupils, it will usually refer to a teacher who has expertise in the field or an educational psychologist who is also a qualified teacher but who has specialist knowledge of the ways in which children learn most effectively.

An Educational Psychologist (EP) is a qualified teacher who, among other skills, has been trained to assess children's special educational needs and make recommendations to meet those needs. Often the EP is the most crucial person involved in children's Stage 3 assessments. The EP is trained to advise on every kind of special educational need. Most schools will especially ask an EP to become involved where children have a behaviour problem or a specific learning difficulty (dyslexia) or a very complex difficulty. The EP will usually assess children in some detail at this stage, often giving them a test of their underlying ability, using what in layman's terms would be called an IQ test. However, the EP will probably be more interested in finding out how well children learn than in giving parents a crude IQ score. The main item in the report should be the recommendations listed for the school to follow.

Learning Support Teacher (LST) These teachers vary by name according to the authority for whom they work, but most LEAs will have at least a Primary Service which offers extra support and teaching to children with SpLD (Dyslexia). Other names you may come across are: peripatetic teachers, teachers from the service for children with specific learning difficulties, special needs team teachers, 1993 Act Teachers and many more.

The specialist teacher will usually have an extra qualification to teach children with special educational needs such as a Diploma or a Master's degree. Ideally they will also have a qualification recognised by the British Dyslexia Association as appropriate for the teaching of dyslexic children. We would issue a minor caution here. An excellent teacher with a dyslexic qualification is the ideal, but an excellent teacher without one will probably be more effective than a weak teacher with the right piece of paper. The qualifications concerned should be approved by the British Dyslexia Association (BDA). There are two levels of approved status from the BDA: ATSBDA means Approved Teacher Status and AMBDA means Associate Member.

Speech and Language Therapist (SALT) Many children with specific learning difficulties have associated or underlying speech and language problems. Where children are seeing a therapist for such problems it is essential that the school and the therapist work together. The knowledge which the school has of children may help the therapist's work and vice versa. In these circumstances, the therapist may well provide an IEP for children and may request that the school reinforce the work being done in the therapy sessions. This is often achieved with a simple language programme which will form part of children's IEPs. For instance, if children are being taught to articulate particular sounds with the therapist, then the school may be asked to assist them when those sounds are used in the classroom. This would be written in the IEP. An example follows:

Target: Will be able to make the sounds 'ch' and 'sh'.

Provision: The teacher will listen for the child's use of the sounds and will prompt the child orally if they are pronounced incorrectly'.

Not all children with SpLD will require help from a therapist. Sometimes children will not be seeing a Therapist but the SENCO may suspect an underlying language difficulty. In these circumstances the SENCO should refer to the therapist for assessment and advice.

Educational Social Worker (ESW) Educational Social Workers have a far wider brief than their popular image as the people who catch truants. They will usually be able to offer parents and school valuable advice on children's emotional well-being. They do encourage children to come to school if they are reluctant and will do more than encourage if the children and their parents do not respond. However, they can also offer services such as counselling or act as an informed link between home and school. Most dyslexic pupils will not need help from an ESW but there are occasions where their services will be crucial. If their help is suggested for children parents should not be put off by the term 'social worker': these teams of professionals are employed by Education Authorities for educational reasons.

If children are placed at Stage 3, it will mean that the school has more serious concerns about their progress. It means they have tried to solve their difficulties on their own and have decided they need more specialist advice and support. You should also be concerned but not over-concerned.

An example of a typical Stage 3 Individual Education Plan is given on the following page. Its main difference to the educational plan prepared for Stage 2 is that it will tend to be more detailed. It will — or should — be based, to a large extent, on the recommendations made by the Stage 3 specialist. The targets will also be similar to those for Stage 2. There will probably, but not necessarily, be more of them and they may be more detailed. Schools and parents need to be sensible here. Too many targets may look impressive but can be counter-productive. By trying to achieve too much, too little may be the only outcome.

Targets may contain jargon or specialist language. If they do and you are not sure what is meant, then ask. A Stage 3 specialist should always offer to see a child's parents and key teaching staff after the assessment. This is to discuss and explain their findings. If this is not offered and you would like the opportunity, then insist on it.

Reviewing progress at Stage 3

So far, reviews will probably have been fairly informal affairs. Usually there would only have been parents, the SENCO and the teacher involved. In these circumstances, the process should be kept fairly low key. Stage 3 reviews are inevitably more formal. The number of people present can increase quite significantly. Here is the **typical membership of a Stage 3 review panel**:

- Headteacher;
- SENCO;
- Class or subject teacher;
- Special Needs Teacher;
- Educational Psychologist;
- Parent(s)/guardian(s);
- The child (if appropriate).

STAGE THREE

I.E.P

Individual Education Plan

Name

Robert Andrew Jones

Age

| 10 | Years | 3 | Months |

Class / Form	**N.C. Yr**	**SEN Stage**	**I.E.P. Date**	**Next Review Date**
Mr S Williams	6	3	29 Sep, 96	Feb 97

Reading Age	8.9
Spelling Age	7.1
Numeracy Age	10.9

Tel 939048390483092

Are parents able / willing to help support at home

○ Yes
○ No

I.E.P. Monitoring by:

☐ Headteacher   ☐ Pastoral Head
☒ SENCO   ☒ Parent
☒ Class teacher   ☒ External Agencies
☐ Subject teacher   ☐ Key Worker

Medical/Pastoral requirements

Robert is asthmatic and needs to use his ventilator occasionally during the school day.

Pen portrait of the pupil

Robert has a very specific difficulty with writing and spelling. In all other areas of the curriculum he is above average.   He has had extra help for several years and appeared to make steady progress but over the last year has stood still. He saw the Educational Psychologist (report 12.6.96) who found he is dyslexic. His IQ score is 139 with very low scores in short term memory and coding. The EP recommended a move to Stage Three. This is his first stage three IEP.

TARGET: It is intended that by the next review adequate progress will enable the pupil to :-	**PROVISION:** The following provision will normally be made available :-	**TARGET ACHIEVED:** with date and/or comment :-
read with fluency his own choice of books from the school library.	Opportunities to read regularly to an adult reader with a view to increasing fluency.	
Will be able to spell the following sight words with 80% accuracy on three consecutive occasions: first 200 McNally/Murray	A programme to develop ability to write words which can be read on sight supplied by the Learning Support Teacher.	
spell simple phonetically plausible monosyllabic words.	A programme to develop ability to read spell simple phonetically plausible monosyllabic words.	
use a spell checker appropriately.	The school will buy a spellchecker and Robert will taught how and when to use it.	
Will consistently write neatly and clearly.	Robert will be encouraged to write more consistently in a clear and legible cursive style.	
proof read writing for spelling errors.	Robert will be expected to proofread his own work and correct errors before a final draft is written.	
plan writing before it is written.	The Learning support teacher in liaison with the classteacher will teach Robert how to plan and structure his writing.	
His inhaler must be readily accessible for him.	Robert will carry his inhaler in his bag. A spare inhaler will be kept in the Secretary's office.	

This review recommends that   Robert will move to Stage Three

Possible outcomes of a Stage 3 Review

Conclusion of review	Possible outcome
The child has made good progress. Targets have been achieved and the difficulties seem well on the way to being resolved.	Return to Stage 2 with an IEP designed to reinforce progress made at Stage 3.
The child has progressed well. This progress seems dependent on the current level of provision.	Continue at Stage 3.
Some progress has been made but there are doubts about the appropriateness of some of the actions recommended by the specialist.	Either the specialist will re-assess the child or another agency might be asked to assess the child.
The child has not made sufficient progress or is falling further behind. The meeting is of the view that the Stage 3 IEP was appropriate to the child's needs. However, the child needs more support than an ordinary school can offer from its own resources.	The school will refer the child to the Local Education Authority for a statutory assessment of his or her special educational needs.

Nature of the Stage 3 Review Meeting

Discussion should again centre on progress towards the targets set within the IEP and the setting of new targets for the next IEP. It will be the aim of all professionals within a meeting to maintain a constructive, mutually supportive level of discussion, seeking at all times to serve the best interests of the child within the constraints under which they all work.

However, despite this positive approach, parents may find that they do not agree with the recommendations of others at the meeting or the conclusions of the meeting as a whole. It can be difficult to maintain their opposition in these circumstances. They may feel a little over-awed by the number of people there, or anxious because they do not fully understand the technical terms or jargon which may be used. When this happens, it is easy either to give in, because the professionals seem so unified in their opinions or to become aggressive for the same reason. If parents suspect that they are going to be in disagreement with the professionals in a proposed meeting they should consider going with someone to support them in putting their point of view. A friend or relation may help. Some LEAs sponsor befrienders to assist parents in these circumstances. When parents or schools are not sure whether their LEA does so they should contact the Special Needs Section and ask. Some independent organisations may also assist. The local branch of the British Dyslexia Association, for example, may provide a befriender. Whatever parents do, there may come a time when, despite the good intentions and professional judgements of all concerned, they still remain unhappy with the review's outcome. We would suggest that, in this situation, they follow these strategies:

State your views coolly and clearly. Make it plain that you do not accept the outcome of the meeting. Ask for a further meeting with the Headteacher to discuss the outcome privately with him or her. Put this view in writing to the Headteacher. If you remain unhappy there are several options open to you, dependent on the nature of your dissatisfaction.

If you believe your child needs a statutory assessment and the meeting does not

If the meeting does not believe your child requires statutory assessment but you do, then you have a right to make the referral yourself directly to the LEA. The LEA will not be obliged to accept the referral. The first thing it will do, on receiving your letter, will be to write to the Headteacher seeking his or her views. Ultimately if the LEA does not accept your referral you have a right of appeal against this decision to the SEN Tribunal. See the next chapter for more on parental rights here.

If you do not believe your child needs a statutory assessment but the meeting does

You cannot prevent the school referring your child. It is the Headteacher's duty to do so if s/he believes that the school is unable to meet your child's needs from within its own resources. However, on receiving the referral from the school the LEA will write to you seeking your views. You should write or phone back carefully explaining your reasons. The LEA may still decide to go ahead with the assessment but it will be extremely reluctant to do so. Our advice is that if you do not persuade the LEA to end the assessment then let it proceed. The assessment itself should only be helpful to your child and the school. If you disagree with its outcome then you have sound rights of appeal against it — although hopefully it will not get that far.

If you wish to have a second specialist opinion but the meeting does not agree

Write to the senior manager of the Service whose second opinion you are seeking. Explain why you wish to have a second opinion. S/he will contact you and probably discuss the matter with you. As long as you can demonstrate that you have a reasonable case then most managers will arrange for a second opinion. If ultimately s/he does not do so and has not persuaded you that one is unnecessary, then write to the Director of Education with your concerns.

If you are unhappy with some aspect of the IEP or its implementation within the school

There are two courses of action open to you here:

(1) The SEN Policy for the school should contain a complaints procedure. Follow that procedure.

(2) The LEA has a duty to monitor special needs provision in its schools. Complain to the Director of Education.

Make sure you do 1 before considering 2.

The next chapter considers in detail what happens if Stage 3 meetings decide that children should be referred for statutory assessment. This assessment will determine if the children's special educational needs are severe enough for the Local Education Authority to make extra provision to meet them.

Summary of Chapter 8

This chapter:

- described how the following parts of the UK Code of Practice for Children with Special Educational Needs apply to dyslexic children:

- the background to the Code;

- the Code's principles and practice;

- schools' Special Needs Policies;

- the role of the Special Needs Coordinator;

- the first three stages of assessmen;

- Individual Education Plans and target setting;

- the roles of the Educational Psychologist, Learning Support Teacher, Speech and Language Therapist and Educational Social Worker.

Chapter 9

Children with Statements

This chapter explains the what, how and why of the statementing procedure. It is based on the Code of Practice for the Identification and Assessment of Special Educational Needs (Sections 3.1 to 6.61) in the UK. It covers the assessment process which may lead to a statement being written. It explains the appeal procedures which can be used if parents are unhappy with an LEA's decisions about a child's statement or need for a statement. During this chapter we stress the importance of cooperative working between all those involved in assessing a child's needs and in subsequent decisions about meeting those needs.

What is a Statement?

Statements of special educational need are intended for a small proportion of children who have special needs. One of the main aims of the statementing process is to sort out those children who require statements from those who do not. In most counties, only children with very significant levels of dyslexia will be 'statemented'. A statement is a legally binding contract made between a child's parents and the Local Education Authority (LEA). Following a detailed assessment, the statement should state all the child's special educational needs and then specify how the LEA will meet them. It should name the school where this provision will be made. It will also identify a child's related non-educational needs and name the other agency (usually the Health Service or Social Services) which will make provision to meet them. A simplified example of a statement is given on the next page. We have omitted some of the standard wording from this example to make it clearer.

A Simplified Example of a Statement

PART 1   THE CHILD'S DETAILS

Name Robert Jones	**Parent's/Guardian's name** Mr and Mrs Jones
DOB 17.7.89	**Address** As for child
Address 4, Parkway, Bilton	**Previous Schools** Parkway Infants

---

PART 2   THE CHILD'S SPECIAL EDUCATIONAL NEEDS

Robert is experiencing significant specific learning difficulties (Dyslexia). Despite appropriate help from his school and his parents, his literacy skills are well below the level which would be predicted by his above average intelligence. He has special educational needs in the following areas:

1.   He needs to improve his reading and skills to a level appropriate to his age and ability.
2.   He needs to improve his short-term memory recall.
3.   He needs to write in cursive style.
4.   He needs to improve his self-esteem and self-confidence.

PART 3   PROVISION TO MEET THE CHILD'S SPECIAL NEEDS

(A)   Objectives for this provision

1.   To accelerate his rate of progress in reading and spelling.
2.   To improve his recall skills.
3.   To develop a cursive style of handwriting.
4.   To improve his self-confidence and self-esteem.

(B)   Provision to be funded by the LEA

1.   He will be taught by a specialist special needs teacher for 3 hours a week in a group of no more than three other pupils.
2.   This teacher will devise an individual educational programme for him to help him towards achieving objectives 1–4.
3.   These programmes will be multi-sensory in nature.
4.   The programmes will be structured, thorough and cumulative.

(C)   Review arrangements

1.   The school will set specific improvement targets for each objective.
2.   The targets will include review dates.
3.   This statement will be formally reviewed within twelve months.

PART 4   SCHOOL WHERE THE PROVISION WILL BE MADE

Parkway Junior School

PART 5   NON-EDUCATIONAL NEEDS

Robert is long-sighted and needs glasses for reading and writing.

PART 6   NON-EDUCATIONAL PROVISION

Robert's vision is reviewed every six months by an optician.

What is the Function of a Statement?

The statementing procedure is part of the Code of Practice for special educational needs. You will recall from Chapter 8 that the Code recommends five stages for the assessment of children with special educational needs. The first three school-based stages were dealt with in that chapter. The final two stages cover the statementing procedure. It is the LEA not the school which has lead responsibility during these stages. It is the LEA which must agree that a child may need a statement, arrange the assessment necessary to see whether a statement is needed, to write one if so, and to fund any extra provision which it specifies.

The main purpose of a statement is to make special educational provision for a child which is over and above that which an ordinary school could be reasonably expected to provide. This needs further explanation. Schools will usually have a proportion of their budget allocated to them specifically to help them make appropriate provision for pupils with special needs. They may use this money in a number of ways. Examples of this are employing a specialist teacher or non-teaching assistant, paying extra responsibility points for a special needs coordinator or buying special books and equipment. However, the funding will not normally be sufficient to meet the educational needs of those children with the most severe levels of learning difficulty. In these cases, where it can be shown that the school cannot reasonably be expected to meet children's special needs, it becomes the LEA's responsibility to do so. The statementing procedure is the process by which this kind of decision is made.

It must again be stressed that statements are only intended for children with the most severe levels of difficulty. Nationally there is an expectation that about 2% of children will have statements. In reality, the percentage varies widely from LEA to LEA. Some LEAs barely issue statements for 1% of their pupils, others for over 7%. The figures for your local authority are publicly available. They have to be published by the Authority each year as one of its Performance Indicators. If you want them, they are available from the LEA or the local library. Be careful though, when interpreting these figures. Although it may look that way, the percentages we quoted here may not mean that the authority statementing only 1% of children makes less provision for children with special needs than the LEA which has statements for 7%. The first LEA may give its schools more money for special needs in the first place or it may fund extra provision for children without the need for statements. The important thing to emphasise at this point is that before a child can be considered for a statement, s/he must be shown to be experiencing a severe level of learning difficulty.

An Overview of Statutory Assessment — the Statementing Procedure

Readers involved with teaching or rearing significantly dyslexic children will need to become very familiar with the statementing procedure. Therefore we intend to deal thoroughly with the subject in this chapter. Statementing's proper title is *'statutory assessment'*. Statementing follows a number of distinct phases. We thought it would be helpful to summarise these in tabular form to give you an **overview of the whole process**. We will then take each phase in turn and explain it in some detail. Children may have statements in both non-maintained and grant-maintained schools. There are slight variations in some procedures for these schools which we do not feel are important enough to warrant separate mention.

Phase	Action	Comment
1	*The School refers the child to the LEA*: following the second or subsequent Stage 3 Review the school believes it is unable to meet the child's needs without extra provision from the LEA. In consultation with the parents and others involved with the child, it refers the child to the LEA for an assessment to see if this is the case. *The parents refer the child*: the child's parents refer the child independently to the LEA for statutory assessment. *The Health Trust or Social Services refer the child*: normally this would only be for a pre-school child.	At this stage, if the child is of school age, the onus is on the school to show it has made appropriate provision at Stages 1–3, that the child has a severe difficulty and s/he has still not progressed adequately.
2	The LEA seeks evidence that the child is likely to need a statement. If the school refers, it seeks evidence from the parents. If the parents refer it seeks evidence from the school.	If the LEA does not find sufficient evidence to support the referral it will decide not to make the assessment.
3	The LEA will coordinate the assessment seeking further evidence from a number of sources.	These sources include the parents, the School, the Health Trust and an Educational Psychologist.

Phase	Action	Comment
4	The LEA will consider the evidence from these sources and decide whether or not a statement is necessary.	If it does not feel a statement is necessary it will issue a 'note in lieu of a statement'. This will define the child's needs with an expectation that provision to meet them will be made by the school. Parents, not schools, may appeal against this decision to the Tribunal.
5	The LEA will issue a proposed statement to the parents. This document will state the child's special needs and specify how they will be met. At this point, if not before, the LEA will also usually identify a 'Named Person' to help parents respond to the statement.	This is for parents to consider before it becomes a final document. Parents will be asked to state their preference for the school where they wish the provision to be made.
6	If the parents agree with the statement it will be issued in its final, binding, form. In many cases negotiations are necessary to sort out details of the statement's contents before a final statement is agreed. The final statement will name the school within which the LEA will make the provision. This provision must then be made by the LEA.	Ultimately, if following negotiations the parents and the LEA do not agree about the statement, then the parents have a right of appeal against the final statement to the SEN Tribunal.
7	The statement will be formally reviewed every year. This is the annual review. A Transition Plan is included in the annual reviews for pupils aged 14+.	Parents will be invited to participate in these reviews.

Time-Lines for Statutory Assessment

The Code lays down a fixed time for each stage of the procedure. The effect of this is that a proposed statement should be produced in 18 weeks and a final statement within 6 months. Prior to this, the time taken to complete statements varied dramatically across the country. At one point, the average time was as much as 18 months.

An LEA's success in meeting these timelines must be published annually as one of its Performance Indicators. The actual figure reported is the Authority's success in producing proposed statements within 18 weeks of the referral being accepted. This may seem a long time but it emphasises the fact that the procedure is not to be taken lightly. It is only intended for children with very severe and potentially long-term difficulties. The **time-lines for completion of statutory assessment** are:

Part of process	Time
To seek parents'/school's views on the referral	6 weeks
To coordinate return of advice	6 weeks
To decide whether or not a statement is needed	4 weeks
To issue a proposed statement	2 weeks
To negotiate and issue a final statement	8 weeks

There are a number of possible exemptions to these timings. For instance, the month of August is, for vacation reasons, not counted at all. This has the effect that any assessment period which includes August may last up to 7 not 6 months. Other exemptions are clearly specified within regulations for the Code and include events like children being seriously ill or parents not being available for a period of time.

Referral for Statutory Assessment

Referral for statutory assessment must be to the Director of Education of the LEA in which children live. It is the responsibility of that LEA to decide whether an assessment is necessary. Parents, but not schools, have a right of appeal against an LEA's decision not to assess and only if they made the referral.

While pre-school children can have statements, we would assume that all dyslexic children will have attended school for some time before a statement is considered. For school-age children, the most usual source of referral for statutory assessment is their school. The other likely source is their parents. Routes for referral are different depending on whether it is parents or school who refer. In essence, if the school refers, the LEA will seek the parents' opinion on the referral. If the parents' refer then the LEA seeks similar views from the school. A referral should never be made by a school without the parents' full knowledge and, hopefully, their consent. It is possible and it may be essential, but it is never desirable for a school to refer without parental consent.

School referrals

Most LEAs issue schools with standard referral forms. Completion of these will give it sufficient information to make a decision as to whether statutory assessment is necessary. The Code of Practice lays down the type of evidence which the LEA will need to make its decision.

Information needed to support a referral should include:

- Why the child is being referred?

- Parental views on the child's needs.

- The child's views, where appropriate.

- Evidence of the involvement of any other agencies.

- Details of efforts to meet the child's needs at Stages 2 and 3.

- Individual educational plans and their reviews.

- The views of anyone else with specialist knowledge of the child.

On receiving this information the LEA must decide if statutory assessment is needed. If it concludes that it is necessary then it must write to inform the parents. It should at the same time give them information on the processes involved and seek their views as to whether the referral is appropriate.

The LEA's letter to parents proposing to assess should:

- Tell parents why the LEA wishes to undertake statutory assessment on their child and what procedures are involved.

- Give them the name of an LEA Officer with whom they can discuss this proposal.

- Tell them they have the right to make representations on the proposal within 29 days.

- Give them information on sources of local and national independent advice.

- Tell them about the role of the 'Named Person' (see p.217).

Parents should reply to this letter within 29 working days or six weeks. This is an early opportunity for them to inform the LEA of their views on their child. We would advise them to use it. Some LEAs will send a structured form to assist parents in responding. In replying, parents should try to be brief and to the point. Some parents send in extremely long letters giving every possible detail about their child. The very busy Education Officer who receives this huge bulk of information is unlikely to be able to absorb it all. We would suggest a reply along the following lines, with the words changed according to the actual circumstances.

Dear Mr Jones,

RE: ROBIN SMITH (23.4.89) 16, Winter Street, Whentner

Thank you for your letter saying you intend to assess my son Robin to see if he needs a statement of special need. I am pleased with this decision. I have been worried about Robin's progress for a long time and am convinced he needs more help than Church Street School can possibly give him. I believe that Robin is experiencing a severe level of dyslexia which is hindering his progress at school. He is becoming very upset about this and as a result is starting to behave badly at times at home and school.

I would be grateful if he could be assessed as quickly as possible so that he can get the extra help he needs quickly. Please write to Mrs Susan Williams for more information on Robin. She has been giving him help at home for the last six months and knows him well. Her address is: 17, Winter Street, Whentner.

Yours sincerely,

Parents should be prompt. The earlier they reply to the LEA, the sooner the assessment can begin.

It is unusual for parents of a dyslexic child to refuse to agree that an assessment should go ahead, but it is not unknown. Some parents do not wish their child to be singled out for extra attention. Some fear that the child might be sent to a special school. A few authorities maintain special schools for dyslexic children but most provide for these pupils with extra support within a mainstream setting. Some parents' main fear, however, is that the child may be sent to a special school for children with more general learning difficulties. This should not happen. It is not appropriate for a dyslexic child.

If parents do not wish the assessment to proceed they should be very clear about their reasons when they reply to the LEA. We would recommend that they ask for a meeting with a representative of the LEA to discuss their concerns face to face. Although it is our understanding that LEAs can proceed with an assessment against parental wishes, most LEAs would be very reluctant to do this. We would strongly recommend that, unless they have strong reasons not to do so, parents agree to it. The statementing process is meant to be in a child's best interests. It should provide parents and schools with a detailed analysis of the child's learning styles, abilities and attainments. If a child needs extra help then it should lead to that assistance being provided.

Parents retain a large degree of control throughout the process. They can be confident that while they may not ultimately get from it as much help for their child as they would like, the LEA is unlikely, for instance, to try to *force* their child to leave their present school to attend another they do not like. The LEA Officer may say that they can only offer the support a child needs in School B. If the parents say they will only accept it in School A, then ultimately negotiations will almost certainly centre not on the LEA forcing a move to School B but trying to *persuade* the parents to accept this move. If the parents continue to refuse it then the child will almost certainly remain in School A. However, the child will probably not receive there all the help that would be available in School B. In this negative sense, parents exercise considerable power over the choice of school for their child. Conversely their ability to force the LEA to offer the necessary support in School A is not great if the LEA believe they can provide it more efficiently in School B. We will cover the right to choose a school later in this chapter.

Parental referrals

We would encourage the idea that all referrals should originate from the school with parent's full consent and involvement. This is for two reasons. Firstly, with a school referral should come sufficient information for the LEA to make a quick decision about the need for assessment. Parents are unlikely to be able to supply this information independently of the school. Secondly, the process is more likely to work well if school and parents are working together and effectively submit a joint referral via the school.

There may arise circumstances where parents will wish to refer independently of the school. There may not be a good working relationship or parents may feel that the school is dragging its feet over their child or that they are not taking their child's difficulties seriously enough. Regrettably some schools may have an inadequate knowledge of the needs of dyslexic children and it is possible that they could underestimate the extent of a child's difficulties. However, the profile of dyslexia is high in most state schools and has been so for some years now. This is largely owing to the work of the British Dyslexia Association, the Dyslexia Institute, pioneering teachers and LEA personnel and the universities. Therefore, today ignorance of dyslexia is rare in most schools. It can still arise though and when it does the capacity for parents to refer directly to the LEA is vital.

The LEA must do a number of things when a parental request is received. As with much of the Code, the language it uses appears to give parents significant rights. When looked at more closely however, those rights are rather frail. This is what the Code says at first:

> parents may ask the LEA to conduct a statutory assessment. The LEA must comply with such a request. (Section 3.17)

That strong word *'must'* sounds very powerful. But it is immediately qualified with the following:

> unless they have made a statutory assessment within 6 months of the date of the request or unless they conclude, upon examining all the available evidence, that a statutory assessment is not necessary.

In reality, it is almost completely up to the LEA whether it decides to make an assessment or not. Of course, parents can appeal to the Tribunal if the LEA refuses to comply with their request, but this can be a very large mallet for such a small nut. At the end of such an appeal, even if it is upheld, the LEA can still conclude, at the end of the subsequent assessment, that a statement is not needed. Despite this reservation, it is our experience that LEAs take parental referrals very seriously. If there is evidence that the child needs assessment it will be arranged.

On the receipt of a parental referral the LEA must:

(1) Contact the child's school to inform them that the parents have made a referral. They should seek information from the school on similar lines to that which would have been provided if the school itself had made the referral.

(2) Contact the parents to:

- ask for more information about their concerns

- see how well they have been involved in the child's special needs provision at school.

- Give them similar information to that which would have been given them if the school referred.

Fast-track referrals

One of the main things an LEA will seek with a referral is to assure itself that proper provision has been made for the child at the earlier stages of the Code. This is to ensure that schools have discharged their responsibilities fully at these stages. Therefore, LEAs will normally insist that Stages 1–3 of the Code have been correctly and fully followed prior to referral. If they have not, they should pass this responsibility back to the school.

However, for a small number of children it may be necessary for the LEA to waive this requirement. The Code allows for this with the so called 'fast-track' procedures. These permit an LEA to accept a referral in exceptional circumstances without the earlier stages having been fully followed. This would not normally be relevant to dyslexic children. These procedures are usually invoked only when children have suddenly developed a significant level of learning difficulty following say, a road traffic accident or a major emotional trauma. However, it can be relevant to dyslexic children in some circumstances.

We can find three reasons for fast-track referrals being accepted for dyslexic children. The first reason is if some form of damage to the brain or nervous system has caused a severe dyslexic condition. Secondly, where children have arrived from another country where the Code does not operate and their needs have not been recognised or appropriately. Thirdly, there is the rare but regrettable situation where children's specific learning difficulties have not been recognised by the school and have been left unattended.

For whatever reason, it seems inevitable that some dyslexic children will have very significant learning difficulties identified at a point when insistence on slavishly following the Code's stages would be wholly detrimental to them. A possible example will illustrate this. An 11-year-old boy was about to transfer to secondary school. He was a quiet, happy child who always appeared simply slow to his teachers. They placed him at Stage 2 of the Code where he remained for years. He quietly plodded along, not making much progress but apparently achieving at his potential. Then he was routinely referred to an educational psychologist. The assessment which followed meant that the school's view of him had to dramatically change. The psychologist found him to have above average general ability but with the reading and spelling ability of an average 5 year old. In this context and similar ones, we would say forget the stages. This child has been in full-time education for 6 years and is virtually illiterate. For now, forget the bureaucracy and get the statementing procedures going so that he can receive some extra help quickly.

If the parents or school or both together feel that the fast-track procedures should be used then they must make representations to this effect to the LEA. In nearly all such cases the LEA will seek advice from the Stage 3 agency involved to see if they agree about the need to speed the procedures up.

Making consistent decisions

The Code tells LEAs that they should make 'consistent judgements' on referrals. The Code itself contains criteria for making these decisions. This includes a section on specific learning difficulties (dyslexia). Many LEAs have found these criteria too broad to help them make consistent decisions and have produced more specific ones of their own. This is an important area which we need to cover in some detail. To begin with the Code's criteria. The following is a summary of the Code's criteria for deciding whether dyslexic children require a statutory assessment:

The child's learning difficulty

There should be evidence of:

- an extreme discrepancy between attainments in different core National Curriculum subjects (English/Welsh, Mathematics, Science). (For instance average levels in Science and Mathematics but significantly lower in English);

- an extreme discrepancy within English/Welsh and Mathematics, e.g. average levels of Speaking and Listening but significantly lower levels in Reading and Spelling;

- mismatch between the child's potential and actual attainments e.g. results of standardised tests of cognitive ability are much higher than the reading or spelling levels which the child attains;

- the child being clumsy, or as having problems with orientation, sequencing, perception and language;

- associated and severe emotional and behavioural difficulties.

The child's special educational provision

There should be evidence that the school has:

- ensured that the whole school is working to offer the child education appropriate to the child's specific difficulties;

- in conjunction with external experts has provided the child with an individual educational plan which is appropriate to the specific nature of the child's difficulties, including multi-sensory strategies and structure reading and spelling programmes;

- provided evidence that the child has not significantly progressed despite appropriate support;

- enlisted the help of parents in delivering the child's educational plan;

- has sought appropriate technological assistance, e.g. spellcheckers, remediative programmes;

- monitored the child's emotional and behavioural responses to the learning difficulty;

- sought medical help if it was appropriate.

Where the balance of evidence presented to and assessed by the LEA suggests that the child's learning difficulties:

- are significant and/or complex;

- have not responded to relevant and purposeful measures taken by the school and external specialists;

- *may* call for special educational provision which cannot reasonably be provided within the resources normally available to mainstream schools in the area.

the LEA should consider very carefully the case for statutory assessment of the child's special educational needs.

It is against these criteria that the Code states LEAs should make their decisions. However, while welcoming them as a first attempt to gain some kind of national consistency in this area, many LEAs have not found them sufficiently precise to guide their own decisions. They ask questions like: What is an extreme discrepancy? What is significant progress? What is an appropriate educational plan? To help answer some of these questions LEAs have designed their own local criteria to enable them to be more objective and consistent in their decision-making. To illustrate this, we now list some criteria for dyslexic children which are being explored by a group of LEAs working together:

Criteria for decisions about statutory assessment for pupils with specific learning difficulties (dyslexia)

General

Some pupils will have considerable difficulties in reading, writing, spelling or numeracy which are not typical of their achievements in other fields or of their general ability. They may be good at developing particular skills and they may possess verbal skills which are far in advance of their reading and writing skills. These difficulties could be connected with problems relating to remembering sequences, coordination difficulties and difficulties with visual and audio-visual perception.

Pupils with specific learning difficulties can feel very frustrated and develop emotional and behavioural problems. The educational psychologist can make an assessment when it is suspected that a child has a specific learning disability. Children not having substantial difficulties will be afforded the relevant assistance from the resources which are normally available to schools.

Action by the school

It is expected that the school will have evidence to demonstrate that it has acted as follows before an application for statutory assessment is considered:

- will have formulated, implemented, monitored, regularly reviewed and recorded Individual Education Plans at Stages 2 and 3;

- will have sought advice from an appropriate external service and will have acted upon it;

- will have sought the opinion of parents/guardians and the child himself/herself where appropriate;

- the parents will have been given every opportunity to participate fully in assisting the school to implement and evaluate the individual education plan;

- will have ensured that the child has access to the curriculum through careful differentiation and by means of supportive teaching, resources and care.

- will have sought, where required, appropriate advice to satisfy any social, emotional or behavioural needs;

- will have investigated the advantages of information technology and, where appropriate, will have ensured that the child has access to suitable equipment.

The criteria

It is determined that evidence exists to make a statutory assessment when, in accordance with results of standardised tests, the difference between achievement and ability is likely to occur 2 out of 100 times or less (see Table). Standardised tests are used in assessing reading and numeracy. We consider that children functioning with a Reading Age of 9:0 years or more are unlikely to need a statutory assessment.

Table of Criteria for pupils with SpLD (Dyslexia)

Age group	Year group	Ability or achievement test	National Curriculum level
7 years old	Y2	A difference between achievement and ability which would be present in only 2% of children of this age.	Working at pre-Level 1 in a specific attainment target (AT)*
8 years old	Y3	A difference between achievement and ability which would be present in only 2% of children of this age.	Working pre-Level 1 in a specific AT*
9 years old	Y4	A difference between achievement and ability which would be present in only 2% of children of this age.	Working within Level 1 in a specific AT*
10 years old	Y5	A difference between achievement and ability which would be present in only 2% of children of this age.	Above Level 2 but lower than expected of children of the same age in a specific AT*

Age group	Year group	Ability or achievement test	National Curriculum level
11 years old	Y6	A difference between achievement and ability which would be present in only 2% of children of this age.	Above Level 2 but lower than expected of children of the same age in a specific AT*
12 years old	Y7	A difference between achievement and ability which would be present in only 2% of children of this age.	Unlikely to achieve Level 3 at the end of Key Stage 3 in a specific AT*
13 years old	Y8	A difference between achievement and ability which would be present in only 2% of children of this age.	Unlikely to achieve Level 3 at the end of Key Stage 3 in a specific AT*
14 years old	Y9	A difference between achievement and ability which would be present in only 2% of children of this age.	Unlikely to achieve Level 3 at the end of Key Stage 3 in a specific AT*

* This only applies to Mathematics or specific attainment targets in English (English medium schools)/Welsh and English (Bilingual schools). For pupils in Bilingual schools it will need to be demonstrated that the child has followed English programmes of study for an appropriate period.

Using the criteria laid down by the Code alongside its own (if devised), the LEA must now decide, using the evidence provided by parents and the school, if a statutory assessment is indicated for children who have been referred.

Saying the LEA makes the decision can be misleading. What actually happens is that representatives of the local Director of Education do the deciding. There is no consistent system across the country for doing this. In some Authorities, an educational psychologist will make this decision. In others it is made by a single specialist officer. However, most LEAs employ a panel of people for this purpose. Typically such a panel would consist of the lead officer for statementing or special needs in the LEA, an educational psychologist, specialist special needs teachers and representative headteachers. Some Authorities also include representative parents.

If it is decided that an assessment is necessary, the LEA will then ask for further information on the child. If an assessment is not felt to be required then it must write to the school and parents saying so and giving their reasons. If the referral was made by parents then they have a right of appeal against it. This appeal is to the SEN tribunal. The appeal process is covered later in this chapter.

Collecting Further Evidence

Having decided to make an assessment the LEA must now arrange to receive further advice on the child. This advice is collected in the form of written reports called Appendices. The term 'appendices' is used because if a statement is issued on the child, the advice will be part of that statement in the form of appendices to it.

Advice-givers have 6 weeks to make any individual assessments necessary, write it up and send it to the LEA. The table summarises the nature of each piece of advice.

Advice which the LEA can seek for statutory assessment

Name of advice	Person or agency responsible	Nature of this advice
Appendix A: Parental Representations	Parents	This is the parents' written response to the LEAs proposal to assess their child at the time of referral.
Appendix B: Parental Evidence	Person or agency requested by the parents	This is advice from other sources which the parents have asked the LEA to seek or which they have provided themselves.
Appendix C: Parental Advice	Parents	This is the parents' own advice.
Appendix D: Educational Advice	The child's school	The school will give details of the child from an educational perspective. National Curriculum achievements, progress at Stages 1–3, the child's relationships with other children and adults are covered. Some LEAs will ask schools to tell them the child's views also.
Appendix E: Medical Advice	This advice is coordinated by the Health Trust	This will give information on any relevant medical condition the child may be experiencing, e.g. for a dyslexic child advice might be sought from a speech therapist or optician.
Appendix F: Psychological Advice	An educational psychologist	Using observation, discussion, testing and other information on the child the Educational Psychologist will give a considered and informed overview of the child as a learner in school. For a dyslexic child the results of a test of cognitive ability would be expected (i.e. the child's IQ). This would be compared to the child's performance in literacy and numeracy. to see if s/he is significantly underachieving. The child's style of learning will be assessed along with social and emotional development. For a dyslexic child this is normally the key piece of advice upon which major decisions about the child will be based.
Appendix G: Social Services Advice	A social worker	If a Social Worker or Educational Social Worker is involved with the child, a written report will be requested.
Appendix H	Various	This is a catch-all section designed to include any advice which the LEA requests that has not previously been covered.

This advice is mainly returned to the LEA in the form of written reports. Some schools and parents also send photographs, audio and video tapes. These can be very useful in filling in the whole picture of the child. They can be difficult to copy for to everyone else involved in the assessment, however.

Using This Evidence to Decide whether a Statement is Necessary

The LEA has 4 weeks to consider this evidence and decide whether a statement is necessary for the child and, if so, what it should contain. Once again, methods for doing so vary widely across the country. Some authorities leave it to one officer or educational psychologist to decide. Increasingly though, as recommended in the Code, LEAs establish Panels similar to those described earlier to make joint decisions.

There is one over-riding factor in deciding if a statement is needed: should it be the school or the LEA which makes the provision necessary to meet the child's needs. The Code gives some clear guidance on this. It says:

(A) **When a statement is not indicated: Provision which should be made by the school**

- Occasional support with personal care from a non-teaching assistant;

- Access to a particular piece of equipment such as a word processor, an electronic keyboard or a tape recorder;

- Minor building alterations such as widening a doorway or improving the acoustic environment;

- Occasional advice from an external specialist.

(B) **When a statement is indicated: Provision which should be made by the LEA**

- Regular direct teaching by a specialist teacher;

- Daily individual support from a non-teaching assistant;

- A significant piece of equipment such as a closed circuit television or a computer with a CD-ROM device with appropriate ancillaries and software;

- A major building adaptation such as the installation of a lift;

- The regular involvement of non-educational agencies;

- Placement in a special school;

- Placement in a special unit attached to a mainstream school;

- Regular significantly disruptive moves of a child with special needs with parents in the Armed Forces.

In other words if a child needs the kind of support specified in (A), then a statement is not normally necessary. If, on the other hand they need type (B) support then a statement would normally be considered necessary.

Some LEAs allocate extra resources to mainstream schools which enable them to make provision for children without a statement which, in other Authorities, would require a statement. This may apply particularly to dyslexic children. Typically, a statement for dyslexic children will provide an extra 1–3 hours of specialist teaching support a week. In some authorities this level of support is provided without the need to go through the statementing procedure. In theory this has many advantages because it saves the time and money involved in making a statement, often estimated in the region of £1000 per child. This is fine in practice providing the extra support is properly managed and monitored so that those children who most need the help actually receive it.

The Note in Lieu

Not all statutory assessments end with statements. In recognition of this the Code introduced the idea of children having a *'note in lieu of a statement'* written on them when the assessment concluded a full statement was not necessary. This means that the LEA has decided a child's needs can reasonably be met from within the school's own resources.

This new and potentially very beneficial development has not received the attention and approval it perhaps deserves. Most parents and schools react adversely to it, often feeling that either the whole process has been a waste of time or that the severity of their child's needs has been underestimated by the assessment. However, the Note in Lieu can be seen very positively. Firstly, it should act as a signal that a child's difficulties are not as severe as previously thought. Parents can be cynical about this suggestion but a professional judgement that a child's needs are less significant than at first perceived should, in theory anyway, be an occasion for relief not cynicism. Secondly, the Note in Lieu is a positive attempt to make full use of all the valuable information which has been gained on a child during the assessment. This should lead to his/her needs being met more effectively within the school.

A Note in Lieu will usually explain to parents why it was decided that a statement was not considered necessary. With it will be copies of the advice on which this decision was based. The Note in Lieu will usually state what a child's special educational needs are and how they should continue to be met. If parents do not agree with this decision, they may appeal against it to the SEN Tribunal. Before doing this, they would be advised to seek a meeting with the Named Officer to discuss the reasons for not issuing a statement and hopefully find a solution satisfactory to them both.

What a Statement Should Contain: The Proposed Statement

If the assessment concludes with a decision that a statement is necessary, it will first be sent to the parents as a draft or proposed document. This proposed statement must conform to the format and contain the information specified in the Code:

Structure and format of a statement

Part	Contents
Part 2 The child's SEN	Details of all the child's special educational needs as identified in the advice
Part 3 Special Educational Provision	**3(a)** A list of the objectives which the provision should aim to meet. **3(b)** The provision required to meet the child's needs and the objectives in 3(a). **3(c)** Arrangements for monitoring progress towards the objectives. These include setting short-term targets and regular review arrangements
Part 4 Placement	The type and name of the school(s) where the provision is to be made
Part 5 Non-educational Needs	All the relevant non-educational needs identified in the advice
Part 6 Non-educational Provision	The provision which the LEA has agreed should be made by the health service or social services

The Proposed Statement should be dated and the Appendices (as described earlier) attached.

The Code also details the information each part of the statement should contain. This is summarised in the table on the next page.

Details of the contents of a statement

Part	Details of information contained
(2) The child's SEN	This should contain: • a description of all the child's needs; • a description of what the child can and cannot do. These needs must be specified. The statement cannot simply say something like 'The needs are identified in the advice.' If the information in the advice conflicts, e.g. If one says the child is dyslexic and the other says he or she is not, then the statement must resolve the disagreement and give reasons for this decision.
(3a) Objectives for the provision	These are the long-term objectives to be achieved by the provision before the statement should be ended, e.g., 'Sarah will be able to read and write at a level which will allow her to cope with these skills in mainstream classrooms.' 'James will be able to write fluently in a cursive style.'
(3b) Provision to meet the objectives	All the provision to meet the child's needs should be set out whether it is to be made by the authority or the school. The LEA remains responsible for arranging all the provision specified. If the provision entails any changes to the child's National Curriculum entitlement these also should be written in. Any special arrangements for external examinations (a statement is not necessary for these arrangements) The provision should be specific, detailed and quantified in terms, for instance of hours of special support. A caveat is added here: 'there will be cases where some flexibility should be retained in order to meet the changing special educational needs of the child.'
(3c) Review and monitoring	This section should state arrangements for setting short-term targets for the child. These relate to the objectives. They are mostly aimed at achievement in one year or from one annual review to the next. They are more specific and more limited than the objectives. For example: 'It is intended that Sarah will improve her measured reading ability by 8 months in the next 12'; 'James will learn how to use a cursive style of handwriting'. Schools, not the LEA, set these targets, within 2 months of the child's placement. The Annual Review will evaluate progress towards the targets and set new ones.

Part	Details of information contained
(4) Placement	This part is left blank in the Proposed Statement. The Final Statement will specify two things: • The type of school: special, mainstream primary, special class in a mainstream secondary and so on; • The name of the school or names if more than one is involved.
(5) Non-Educational Needs	This will set out all the non-educational needs which the LEA proposes to meet or which it has agreed will be met by another agency.
(6) Non-Educational Provision	This specifies the provision to meet the needs identified in Part 5. Objectives should also be specified.

The Proposed Statement will be sent home with a number of other documents:

Papers which should accompany the proposed statement

(A)   An explanatory letter.   This should tell parents that they have 15 working days in which to make representations to the LEA on the statement and that they may *require* a meeting to be held with an officer of the LEA to discuss it.

(B)   Copies of all the advice.   These will be attached as Appendices.

(C)   A formal document called 'Schedule Part A: Notice to Parent'.   This stipulates parents' rights of stating a preference of school in which the special provision should be made. It also tells parents how they can appeal against the final statement.

(D)   Two lists of schools.   The first list is of all the special schools in the Authority's area including independent and grant-maintained schools. The second list is of all the independent schools in England and Wales which have been approved by the Secretaries of State as being appropriate for statemented children.

A copy of the proposed statement should also be sent to every agency or individual who sent advice on the child.

Parental Response to a Proposed Statement

This is probably the part of the process where parents will play their most important role. Although they may fear otherwise, LEA officers will invariably wish to secure the best provision they can for the children for whom they are responsible. However, they may be constrained by financial demands. They must also treat all children fairly and equitably. If children have similar special needs, then they should be allocated similar resources to meet those needs.

Parents do not have the same constraints. At any one time they have the one child to take into account. They know this child better than anyone else. They care about that child more than anyone else. No-one else will fight harder for him or her. In this context the Proposed Statement is vital. It is the LEA's considered declaration as to how much of the special educational cake is to be allocated to their child. Parents therefore need to reflect very carefully on its contents. If they have concerns, we would recommend that they assess the statement using the following checklist or something like it. This can then be taken to any meeting with the LEA Named Officer as a basis for discussion.

In most cases this will not be necessary. Where the school, the assessing agencies and the LEA have worked closely together, before and during the assessment, it is likely that a degree of trust has developed between them. In these circumstance parents may well already be familiar and happy with the contents of the proposed statement before it comes home. For them it may not require more than a careful perusal to ensure that what has been verbally promised is actually specified. They will also need to check that there are no glaring errors or omissions. In other circumstances, or if parents simply wish to get complete clarity about the contents of the statement, some kind of structured response to the LEA is recommended.

Checklist for the proposed statement

Item

Is the basic information in Part 1 correct?

Are the descriptions of needs adequate/accurate?

Is there anything in Part 2 which needs further explanation?

Is there anything in Part 2 with which you disagree?

Are the objectives in Part 3a appropriate to the child's needs?

Is the provision described in part 3b sufficiently specific, detailed and quantified?

Does Part 3b provide for enough extra support?

Item

Is the school's role clearly specified in Part 3b?

Does Part 3b make satisfactory (if any) arrangements for the child's entitlement to the National Curriculum?

Are the arrangements for monitoring and review in Part 3c clear and acceptable?

Are all the relevant non-educational needs identified in the advice included in Part 5?

Does Part 6 make it clear what provision is to be made and by whom?

Is there anything else you would like to raise with the Named Officer?

The Code also lays down timelines for meetings between parents and the LEA to discuss the contents of a proposed statement:

Time-lines for meetings with the LEA

Parents may make representations about the statement within 15 days of its receipt and require a meeting with an LEA officer to discuss it. Within a further 15 days of the meeting they may make further representations or require further meetings with 'appropriate people in the LEA' to discuss the advice given. Within final 15 days from the last meeting they can make further comments to the LEA.

The Named Person

Parents may feel that they need support to negotiate with the Named Officer. The needs of dyslexic children and the provision necessary to meet those needs can be complex. Unless they know of someone personally who can do this, there are two main sources of advice and guidance for parents in this situation. These are the Named Person provided for in the Code and the local branch of the British Dyslexia Association. A contact number for the latter is included in the list of useful addresses.

The Named Person is someone who can inform and support parents about children's special educational needs. The Code says that the LEA must inform parents of the identity of a Named Person at least by the time the Final Statement goes home. Most authorities provide this information well before the Final Statement and at least by the Proposed Statement, the time when it is probably most important that one is available. This is what the Code says about the role of the Named Person:

> The Named Person should be someone whom the parents can trust. He or she should be capable of giving parents accurate information and sound advice. (Section 4.72)

Many Named Persons are reluctant to give advice. They are afraid that they might leave themselves open to legal action if that advice could subsequently be shown to have been detrimental to a child's interests. The role is developing into one of support and information. Most Named Persons will supply parents with the information they need to make a decision and support them in implementing that decision. They will not make the decision for them.

A Named Person can literally be anyone from the next-door neighbour to a national specialist. Many LEAs have made arrangements with other organisations to supply Named Persons for them. For instance, some North Wales Counties have an agreement with the local Citizens' Advice Bureaux to provide them with Named Persons. This is a very successful scheme, much appreciated by the parents who have used it. Elsewhere in Wales many counties use an organisation called 'SNAP' ('Special Needs Advice for Parents').

Although this is usually done in conjunction with the LEA, parents may nominate their own Named Person. Unless parents approach someone who is a known specialist in the field they are unlikely to find someone with a great deal of knowledge about dyslexia. However, most Named Persons take the attitude that if they do not know the answers to your questions then they will find someone who does. Owing to its specific nature, a knowledge of dyslexia and its educational implications is often central to any useful discussion about a child's needs. Therefore, in this area, perhaps more than some others, parents will need specialist information.

Parents and teachers should be clear about the difference between roles of the Named Person and the Named Officer:

> **Named Officer** — employed by, and with allegiance to, the LEA to negotiate statement provisions with parents and schools.

> **Named Person** — independent of the LEA, a source of information and support for parents in their negotiations with the Named Officer.

Naming a School

Chapter 10 describes the range of special education provision potentially available for dyslexic children.

With the Proposed Statement will come a request for parents to state their preference for the school where the statement's provisions will be made. At first sight, this seems to be a significant right for parents. They will have received, during the assessment process, much information to help them decide a preference including the following sources of information:

(a) a list of all the provision made by the LEA for children with special educational needs;

(b) a list of all the area's mainstream schools;

(c) a list of approved independent schools which make provision for statemented pupils.

Together, these lists make an impressive collection of schools; from the local primary to some rather expensive private schools at the other end of the country. Major rights seem to have been given to parents here. But the small print of the Code has hidden meanings which would be better expressed in capital letters. This is what the Code says:

> Parents may express a preference for the school in the maintained sector they wish their child to attend, or make representations for a placement outside the maintained sector. LEAs must comply with a parental preference unless the school is unsuitable to the child's age, ability, aptitude or special educational needs, or the placement would be incompatible with the efficient education of the other children with whom the child would be educated, or with the efficient use of resources. (p. 90)

Similarly later the tone of the Code is strong in language but weak in effect:

> The LEA have a duty to name the parents' preferred school in a statement *so long as the preferred conditions . . . apply: the placement must be appropriate to the child's age, ability, aptitude and special educational needs, while also compatible with the interests of the other children in the school and with the efficient use of the LEAs resources.* (Code of Practice 4.56)

These 'preferred' conditions give an LEA considerable scope to find grounds not to comply with the parents' preferences should they wish not to do so. The Code is saying that usually the LEA will be able to place children where it wishes as long as it can demonstrate the placement is appropriate to meeting their needs. Despite this imbalance of power, in nearly all cases LEAs and parents manage to amicably agree a school between them. Often a change in school is not discussed for dyslexic children. Instead, negotiations centre around the kind and amount of support which will be offered within the child's present school.

To sum up, negotiations over the proposed statement are central to the assessment procedures. The contents of this document are likely to drive children's special education into the near future. It is essential that it comes as close as possible to specifying all of their needs and makes appropriate provision to meet those needs. In many cases the main contents of the statement will be known and accepted by the parents before it even comes home. Parents should carefully check the wording of the statement. They might wish to seek independent advice on it. If there are any problems with its contents then they should seek a meeting with the Named Officer to discuss them. The Code lays down guidelines for these meetings. In most cases, agreement is reached on the statement at this stage. All that remains then is for the LEA to issue a final statement which will confirm that agreement with the parents. Then the provision can begin.

Whatever the difficulties, however wide the gap between themselves and the parents, most LEA officers will seek to arrive at some form of compromise agreement, which is acceptable to both parties. Ultimately, however, if they cannot agree then, there will be no other option but to issue the final statement and for parents to appeal against it. Appeals can only be made against final statements.

The Final Statement

The final statement is exactly what its name suggests: the LEA's last word on the child's needs. This sounds very rigid. In reality, if parents or schools discover a serious error of fact in the final statement or its wording does not reflect the agreements which appeared to have been reached, then most LEAs would be willing to amend it. The statementing process is about people trying to work together in the best interests of the child. For the LEA this wish is tempered by the inevitable constraints imposed by finite budgets and the principle of equal access to funding for all children with special needs.

Unlike the wording in some parts of the Code of Practice, statementing need not be about sticking rigidly to this or that routine, this or that deadline. The professionals involved are nearly in their posts because they have an affinity for children with learning difficulties. Although some may give this impression, most of these officers have no wish to dig their heels in and use bureaucratic niceties to get their own way for the sake of it and to the detriment of the child. With give and take and understanding on both sides, reasonable agreements should be and are reached for the vast majority of children.

There will always be a small minority for whom this does not prove possible. The appeal procedures are in place for this eventuality. With the final statement should come a letter which informs parents of their rights of appeal to the Special Educational

Needs Tribunal (SEN Tribunal). The identity of a Named Person for the child, to support the parents, must also be sent to them, if one has not been agreed already.

The Appeal Procedures

The LEA should give parents full information on their rights of appeal. Some will automatically enclose a booklet from the Tribunal on the appeal procedures. Most will tell parents that this booklet exists and will offer to send it to them if they are considering appealing. Parents **may appeal on the following grounds:**

- The description in Part 2 of the child's special educational needs

- The description in Part 3 of the provision to meet those needs.

- The type and name of school specified in Part 4.

Parents may not appeal against the contents of Parts 5 and 6: non-educational needs and provision. They can appeal against a decision to place in Parts 5 and 6 provision which they believe should be in Parts 2 and 3.

An appeal must be lodged with the SEN Tribunal within 2 months of the parents receiving the statement. The Tribunal is strict on its deadlines. Parents appeal via a standard form. This will ask them to state their grounds of appeal. It is important that all the grounds of appeal are stated at this point. New ones cannot be added later. The process of appeal is the same, whatever point of the process is involved. The Code itself admits that going to appeal can be stressful for parents and time-consuming for the LEA officers concerned. In reality, it can also be stressful for the officers and time-consuming for parents. If possible, it is best avoided. How difficult the process of appeal becomes depends on the relationship which has developed between officers and parents. Some appeals occur in circumstances where, despite the parents and the officers working closely together, an agreement could not be reached. Appeals in these circumstances can be conducted in an almost friendly atmosphere, with each party taking the view that they simply could not agree about the statement and are amicably seeking arbitration to resolve it. Others appeals are vitriolic, angry, venomous affairs where, whatever the outcome, neither party and particularly the child concerned, really win.

Within LEAs, the Tribunal itself has a reputation for being more positive to parents than to LEAs. This is not wholly borne out by the actual figures. The Tribunal regularly publishes the outcomes of its hearings. The most recent summaries indicate that, on the whole, Tribunals involving dyslexic pupils find approximately 50% of cases in favour of parents and 50% in favour of LEAs. Hopefully this means that both parties are given a fair hearing in Tribunals leading to even-handed judgements.

Each Tribunal usually consists of three people: a Chair who will have a legal background, a lay-person with some interest or knowledge in the field and a professional person with considerable knowledge and experience in the education of children with special educational needs . Proceedings are minuted. There is no set format for the hearings. It depends on the Chair. Sometimes each side presents its case, followed by questions from the other side, with a final summing up session each. Other Chairs ask each side to speak specifically to the issues which are central to that case. A decision is not given at the time. It is sent by letter. The findings of the Tribunal can only be contested on points of procedure. The judgement itself cannot be appealed against.

Parents considering appealing should not be put off by the process. The capacity to appeal is an essential right. The field of special educational needs is complex. It does not have a huge body of knowledge over which everyone agrees. Inconsistent and plain wrong decisions can be made by the most well intentioned of LEA officers. An experiment was conducted recently where different LEA officers were given the same evidence collected for a number of different children's statement assessments. They were then asked to produce a statement for each child. The contents of the statements for the same children varied enormously. In the most dramatic example, one person said the child concerned did not need a statement, whilst another would have sent the child to a very expensive, specialist school.

Providing all the people involved treat everyone else with respect, the appeal procedures need not be so traumatic. Initiating an appeal does not mean that it must end up in a Tribunal. Parents and LEAs are encouraged to seek a solution while they are waiting for the Tribunal to be held. This waiting can take several months. Often the nearness of a pending appeal can sharpen minds and make both parties keener to sort it out between themselves. The Tribunal appears to encourage such last minute moving together. They, like everyone else involved, are only interested in reaching solutions which are fair to children

Annual Reviews

Every statement must be reviewed annually on or before the date of the statement or the last review. The main function of the annual review should be to consider a child's progress against the targets which were set 12 months before. The review should consider the following questions:

Main questions to be raised at the annual review

- What are the parent's views on progress on the targets?
- What is the child's view?

- What is the school's view?

- What are the views of anyone else involved with the child?

- Have there been any significant changes in the child's circumstances which affect development or progress?

- Is the current provision appropriate to the child's needs?

- Does the child still require a statement. If not, why not?

- If the child does still require a statement:

- What should the next set of targets be?

- Does the statement need amending?

- Is any further action needed and if so by whom?

The Code lays down the following fixed procedure for the annual review procedure. It is mainly school based with the LEA retaining oversight and involvement where appropriate.

Annual review procedures

(1)   The LEA must give the school 2 months' notice of pupils who require an annual review. They should state who should be invited to the review meeting.

(2)   The Headteacher must request written advice from the key people involved in implementing the statement including the parents.

(3)   The Headteacher must set a date for the meeting.

(4)   The Headteacher must circulate to all those invited to the meeting any copies of written advice. This should be 2 weeks before the meeting.

(5)   The Headteacher or a designated teacher should chair the meeting.

(6)   The meeting should address and answer the previously listed questions.

(7)   The Headteacher must prepare a report summarising the meeting and circulate it to all concerned.

(8)   The LEA must then review the statement in the light of the report.

(9)   If the LEA amends the statement it must send the new version to parents, who have rights of negotiation over its contents which are similar to the initial statement.

(10) Ultimately parents may appeal to the SEN Tribunal against the contents of the revised statement.

The annual review procedure is probably not as well advanced over the UK as a whole as it deserves to be. Practice varies widely, often down to individual school level. Two schools geographically next to each other might have a completely different attitude to the process, one diligent and conscientious, the other regarding the whole affair as rather cumbersome and bureaucratic.

This is unfortunate. Each annual review, and especially the first one, is of equal importance as the original statement. In one way, the first review of a statement is more important than the statement itself. However well informed and intentioned children's first statements might be, they must, to some extent, be a step in the dark. However good the teacher assigned to the child may be, however excellent the reputation of the school, no-one can guarantee that the child will progress as anticipated. The first annual review is an opportunity to gauge how effective the statement's provisions have actually been for him/her. It deserves taking very seriously.

Parents should approach a child's review with care. They should receive the reports to be discussed before the meeting and have an opportunity to digest their contents and seek advice on them. They should be given every chance to express their viewpoint at the meeting. The child's views, especially those of older children, should also be given considerable weight.

The Transition Plan

Prior to the Code being published, all children with a statement were fully reassessed during Year 9. The Code abolished this requirement. Instead it introduced a requirement that each annual review after a child's 14th birthday must include a Transition Plan. As its name suggests, this plan is concerned with a child's transition from school to post school, be that into work or further education. It follows a similar process to the annual review but it asks an additional set of questions. **The key questions for the transition plan for dyslexic pupils are:**

(1) What are the child's curricular needs during the transition years? E.g. Does he or she need dispensation for GCSE examinations?

(2) How are the professionals involved going to plan together for the child's transition?

(3) Which new professionals (i.e. careers, college link persons) need to be involved?

(4) Is there a need for special technological support during and after transition?

(5) Is education after the age of 16 appropriate? If so, where?

(6) What are the parents' adult life expectations of the child?

(7)   How can parents help the child achieve these expectations?

(8)   What information does the child need to make informed choices?

(9)   How can the child contribute to his or her own transition plan?

(10)   What are the child's own expectations and how can these be met?

The main responsibility for coordinating Transition Plans lies with the LEA. An LEA officer should call the meeting and record its outcomes in the form of a plan. While for many statemented children, Social Services and the Health Trust will have a major role to play in their Plan, the involvement of these agencies with dyslexic children is less frequent. For them, the key players in the Transition Plan will usually be the school itself, the careers officer, the educational psychologist and link persons with local Colleges of Further Education which may offer specialist support for dyslexic youngsters on their chosen courses.

The Transition Plan is a new concept. Some LEAs have made rapid strides to ensure that this service is provided at a high level for their pupils. Others have moved less swiftly. The Code does not allow for this variation. Transition Plans are compulsory. Parents can and should insist on their full and proper implementation.

Summary

In theory, the Code of Practice lays down a set of principles and procedures which should ensure that all children will have their special educational needs identified early, and provided for appropriately according to their type and severity, so that progress is maximised. The reality may be quite different. The Code applies to scores of individual LEAs, all with their own priorities and their own interpretations of its requirements. It also applies to many thousands of individual schools, each of whom will implement it differently. Within the schools it applies to hundreds of thousands of teachers, each with their own particular knowledge, experience and tolerance level of children with special needs. These teachers are responsible for the education of millions of children with special needs. Some of these needs will be major, some minor. Some children will respond wonderfully well to extra help, some will reject it out of hand. In the majority of cases, their parents will be passionate advocates of their child's needs and rights.

The Code of Practice attempts to touch a massive number of lives, and tries to impose a structure on an educational establishment and culture which has always been very independent and individualistic. Tell a British teacher that all children in France have the same lesson at the same time every day in school and they recoil in horror. It is no wonder then that the law says that schools must have regard for the Code, rather than say they must follow it precisely as it is laid down.

Despite this reservation, the Code gives children and parents significant new powers, rights and responsibilities. It may use the words 'must have regard', but this is widely interpreted as meaning that schools must have something as good in place, even if they are not following the Code's actual models of practice themselves. Schools and LEAs must be able to demonstrate good practice for their pupils with special needs. Parents should be aware of the Code's new emphasis on their right to insist that their child's special needs are properly identified, assessed and met. That is what the Code is largely about: empowering and informing parents, informing and guiding schools. The best guarantee that these new rights will be protected is for parents themselves to insist on them.

Summary of Chapter 9

This chapter:

- depicted what a statement is and what it is supposed to do;

- gave an overview of the statutory assessment process which can lead to a child having a statement;

- listed the time-lines within which statements should be processed;

- showed how children can be referred for a statutory assessment;

- illustrated the contents of a statement;

- covered the statement appeal and Tribunal process;

- described annual reviews of statements and Transition Plans for children aged 14+.

Chapter 10

Provision for Dyslexic Children

This chapter covers the range of provision available for dyslexic children in state or maintained schools including grant-maintained schools. It begins by describing the continuum of provision which should match the continuum of dyslexic children's difficulties. Finally it takes each stage of the Code of Practice in turn and gives examples of the range and kind of provision which is appropriate for each stage.

Introduction

In Chapter 2 we stated that dyslexia exists on a continuum. This continuum starts with children who have mild difficulties, moves on to those whose problems are moderate and ends with those whose dyslexia is severe. It is logical to assume that the more severe a child's needs are, the more support s/he will need to overcome them. It follows that the continuum of dyslexia should be mirrored by a continuum of provision: the greater the difficulty, the greater the support needed. This continuum is itself matched by the stages of the Code of Practice which we covered in Chapters 8 and 9. You will remember there are 5 stages. Children with the least needs are at Stage 1 and children with most needs at Stage 5. Linking this to our dyslexia continuum, Stage 1 would be equivalent to children with mild difficulties, Stage 3 to moderate and Stage 5 to severe difficulties. We have shown how these all link together in the diagram on the next page.

Typical Provision Made for Dyslexic Children at Each of the Stages

Each stage is now taken in turn. The typical range of support which could be provided at each stage is described. It is important to emphasise that the kind of provision made available varies widely from county to county and from school to school. It is impossible to say that one form of provision is better than another. There is no definitive research in this area; there are no definite answers. So much depends on the nature of the individuals involved.

Is quality of teaching and learning the main factor?

- A brilliant teacher may get better results with a poor programme of work than a poor teacher with a brilliant programme;

A continuum of need and provision

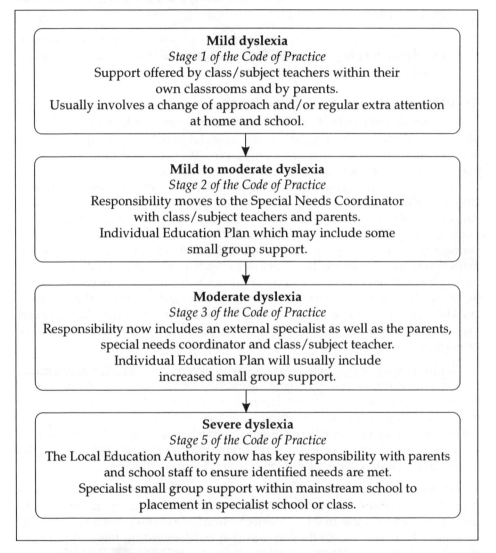

Mild dyslexia
Stage 1 of the Code of Practice
Support offered by class/subject teachers within their
own classrooms and by parents.
Usually involves a change of approach and/or regular extra attention
at home and school.

Mild to moderate dyslexia
Stage 2 of the Code of Practice
Responsibility moves to the Special Needs Coordinator
with class/subject teachers and parents.
Individual Education Plan which may include some
small group support.

Moderate dyslexia
Stage 3 of the Code of Practice
Responsibility now includes an external specialist as well as the parents,
special needs coordinator and class/subject teacher.
Individual Education Plan will usually include
increased small group support.

Severe dyslexia
Stage 5 of the Code of Practice
The Local Education Authority now has key responsibility with parents
and school staff to ensure identified needs are met.
Specialist small group support within mainstream school to
placement in specialist school or class.

- Children may make more progress with an excellent teacher for 2 hours a week than with a poor teacher for 4 hours.

- When both have received the same amount and kind of support, a well motivated and hard-working child will make more progress than an indifferent and idle child.

- Children with supportive and sympathetic parents will progress better with the same amount of support than those whose parents are negative or do not get involved.

- For social reasons, children sent away from home to a special residential school may not progress so well there as children allowed to stay at home and attend their local school with less help.

The philosophy behind the Code's stages

Before we go through the five stages we need to explain a little about the philosophy behind them. Making special provision for children can be disruptive to their overall education and can affect their self-esteem. The extra help arranged for them may be a source of stigma. For instance, taking children out of their mainstream classes to attend a small special help group might improve their reading but it could adversely affect their self-esteem or their social standing in class. Evidence seems to suggest that the older children are the more likely they are to resent being singled out in this way. Younger children seem less affected. However, a large minority of younger children are very resentful of it. Providing children with extra help in the mainstream class can single them out just as much as taking them out of the class. Giving them different work to their classmates will not go unnoticed. Children quickly pick up the hidden messages, however well disguised they are by the teachers. They are often less than sympathetic to the needs of others and can be very cruel to their peers whose difficulties are made obvious by the special help arranged to meet them.

Children for whom the help is arranged can also receive unfortunate messages from it. They can easily assume that it means they are slow or of low ability. If they believe this they may live up to that label and act as though they lack intelligence or motivation when, in fact, they are bright and keen. Added to this, if children leave the class for extra help they will be missing out on what the other children are doing. They may fall behind in that lesson. In other words, while special needs help may be beneficial to children there is a hidden cost to it for many of them.

So the first principle is that the child's education should be affected as little as possible. Extra help should be restricted to the minimum necessary for the child to make sufficient progress. In this context, children have to show that they definitely need the help. Unfortunately the only way they can demonstrate this is by failing to progress with the educational programme being offered to them in the mainstream class. It is a classic 'Catch 22' situation.

That leads to the second, mostly unspoken principle of the Code's stages. This is that the special provision made available for children must be shown to have failed at one stage before they can go on to the next. We have put it this way round rather than say the child must fail before anything can done because this is the emphasis we wish to make: blame the programme not the child. It may come to the same thing, however. The Code of Practice operates on the principle that children must fail at one stage before they go on to the next. This sounds rather cruel, but often seems inevitable. A typical progression through the stages would be like this:

Jenny goes through the first two stages of the Code of Practice

Stage 1:   Jenny is at the beginning of her second term in Year 2. Her teacher is worried that, unlike most of her classmates, she has not picked up the basics of reading. She discusses this with the Special Needs Co-ordinator. They agree that Jenny could be developing a reading problem. They meet with her parents and all agree that they will give Jenny extra attention for her reading over the next term. Her teacher will hear her read at least three times a week and her parents agree to her read at home every night. She is placed at Stage 1 of the Register. A review meeting is called for the last week of term.

At this meeting it is clear Jenny is still not progressing. It is agreed to change her to a new set of reading books which are more finely graded. The teacher will increase the time she spends with her and her parents will encourage her to read once at the weekends as well as during the week. A new review is set for the end of the next term. At this meeting it is evident that Jenny has again not responded. It is agreed that she should move to Stage 2 with a review set for the end of the next term. *She moved to this stage because the support she had been offered had failed to help her make the progress desired of her at Stage 1.*

Stage 2:   Jenny is now at the beginning of Year 3. In consultation with parents and her new classteacher, the Special Needs Coordinator draws up an individual education plan for her. This provides the following for her:

Provision	*Targets*
(1) 30 minutes a week with the special needs teacher to work on high-frequency words and some simple phonic skill	(1) To know by heart the first 20 high-frequency words.
(2) A brief daily reading session with the classteacher.	(2) To know sounds made by two consonants blended together (e.g. fr, tr and so on).
(3) Five sessions of paired reading with her parents each week.	(3) To be able to read independently Book 6 of her reading scheme.

At the next review she has not reached these targets. She has only learnt ten high-frequency words, she struggled reading the book independently and although she could 'read' the blended letters, she tended not to use this skill to help her read. As a result of this meeting, her time with the special needs teacher is increased by 15 minutes a week. Her parents will maintain the paired reading and also agree to give her regular practice with the skills she is learning from the special needs teacher. The classteacher will continue the daily reading sessions and look for every chance to reinforce the special needs teacher's work. It was decided to keep the same targets. Her second Stage 3 Review is held at the end of the next term. At this meeting her teacher reports that she has still not reached the targets. Her work in other areas of the curriculum seems fine. She is a bright child who appears to understand and follow her lessons with ease. Reading is a specific difficulty for her. *Once again the provision made available for her at this stage has failed to help her make sufficient progress. Therefore it is decided to move her to Stage 3 and seek specialist advice.*

If the support provided for Jenny at Stage 3 again did not help her make appropriate progress, then she might need to be considered for a statement at Stage 4. This is how the Code's stages work. They are based on the need to demonstrate that what has been provided at the previous stage has proved inadequate to meet a child's identified needs. Some parents and teachers are baffled by this necessity for children to be seen to fail before extra help can be provided for them at a higher stage. They say: 'Surely it is better for the help to be put in before they fail?'

It is a chicken and egg situation which goes something like this. If children are given extra help before they develop a problem they might not develop it. If they do not develop it then no-one would have known they would have had a problem if the help had not been given. The same dilemma applies at each stage. Many children who are identified at Stage 1 are given a little extra attention and overcome their difficulties quickly. Of those that do not and proceed to Stage 2, most will progress quite happily with that level of extra help. This must be the right way to proceed if resources to meet children's needs are in short supply. By concentrating on children who are demonstrating that they are having difficulties, the Code's procedures ensure that available resources are targetted on those children who need them most.

This means that the Code's procedures are not preventative. They are reactive. They do not seek to stop problems developing but to solve them as they arise. The real answer for most children would be to pour extra resources into the education of very young children at the time when they are being taught to read and write. Small, superbly equipped and expertly taught infant classes would probably stop a large number of literacy difficulties ever arising. The expertise is there already in most infant classes. Small numbers and superb equipment is not.

Provision Linked to the Stages

The next part of this chapter consists of a series of tables, each of which lists the kinds of provision which can be made for children at each stage of the Code. It is important to see these provisions as often being cumulative. Thus, if at Stage 1 parents agree to hear children read at home, then that support will probably be continued at Stage 2. If the school were providing an hour's extra tuition for a child each week at Stage 3 and the statement at Stage 5 funded 2 hours, then the child should also continue to receive the school's original hour.

In each table we list the typical range of extra provision which could be made at each stage with an example of it being used in practice. There are many other examples we could have chosen.

Stage 1: Children with mild difficulties

At this stage the main responsibility lies with the class or subject teacher in consultation with the parents and special needs coordinator. Provision is low key, usually involving minor adaptations to the curriculum or extra individual attention from the teacher and/or parents.

Kind of provision	Example
A small amount of daily attention from the class or subject teacher. This would be for a child who is beginning to slip behind peers in reading aloud or who constantly mis-spells certain words or a secondary school child who has difficulty grasping new concepts.	A brief one-to-one reading session each day in class. The teacher chooses words from the child's writing to be practiced. Subject teachers agree to give the child a little extra explanation when introducing new concepts or skills.
Change or adapt the method or materials. This would be for the child who is not responding to the class reading scheme or who has good phonic skills but has great difficulty learning high-frequency words by sight.	Change to a different reading scheme. Use non-scheme books. Emphasise the initial letter sounds of the words as an aid to memory.
Increase expectations of child. i.e. When a child appears able but this ability is not reflected in the work produced.	The teacher sets targets for the child to achieve. The results are fed back to parents with agreed rewards if they are reached.
Parents working with child at home. This might be helpful when the child needs more reading practice than the teacher can give or the child does not appear to value reading.	Parents agree to hear child read at home each school-day. Parents read to child, read themselves, take child to library, join themselves.

Stage 2:   Children with mild-to-moderate difficulties

At this stage the key responsibility for ensuring children's needs are met lies with the special needs coordinator and class/subject teacher working together and with the parents. An Individual Education Plan should be drawn up, implemented and regularly reviewed.

Kind of provision	Example
Limited withdrawal for regular support in a small group from a designated special needs teacher. Usually the amount of time will be quite small, perhaps only half an hour a week.	Weekly half session improving phonic skills, number bonds or letter formation. The lessons would emphasise multi-sensory teaching.
Limited regular support from another teacher in the mainstream classroom. Time will be quite limited. More frequently used at secondary school than primary, the support teacher will give assistance to children in understanding the lesson.	The support teacher will attend a Year 8 Geography lesson to help pupils complete written tasks.
Support from a Learning Support Assistant (LSA) in the mainstream classroom. (Some schools will fund an LSA to provide 'an extra pair of hands' for classes where there are large numbers of children with special needs. This kind of support will be targeted on children who are struggling to show their real knowledge when recording their work.)	The LSA attached to an infants' class might be asked to focus on the children who have literacy difficulties. At secondary school the LSA might be allocated to children in lessons where there are known to experience most difficulty.
Assessment and monitoring by the SENCO.	It is the responsibility of the SENCO to check on the progress of children at this stage. S/he may delegate this responsibility to other teachers.
Curriculum materials adapted by or under the guidance of the SENCO. This will be needed when children find the reading material in some lessons well above the level of their own reading ability.	Some SENCOs, especially at secondary school will work with other departments to adapt the materials used in lessons to better suit the needs of dyslexic pupils. For instance the language might be simplified or diagrams might be inserted to make the lesson content clearer.
Helping children with concepts and skills which they will be encountering in future lessons. This kind of support may be required when children encounter problems understanding new concepts, especially in subjects like mathematics or languages.	The subject teacher will need to inform the SENCO when these new concepts/skills are to be introduced, The SENCO can then work with the child so that s/he goes into that lesson well prepared.

Kind of provision	Example
Advice on programmes, materials and methods from a specialist teacher. As we have stated before: 'If the child is not learning, change the teaching.' The SENCO may be able to advise non-specialist teachers on the kinds of methods and materials most suited to a particular child's learning styles.	Advice could be given to use lots of concrete examples to instil number concepts or change the reading scheme to one where there are more books at each level.
Programmes for class devised by the SENCO or special needs teacher.	The SENCO may be able to provide the class teacher with programmes which the child can follow in class.
Follow-up work for mainstream class from the special needs teacher.	Similar to the preceding item. It is useful for the special needs teacher to leave the child with work which can be completed back in the mainstream class. This will not only help the child but will also let the mainstream teacher know the kind of work which is being used by the other teacher.

Stage 3: Children with moderate difficulties

Responsibility is now shared between the school, parents and the specialist called in to assess the child and offer advice and guidance. By now a child's difficulties are acknowledged to be more serious and to require more of the school's time and attention. One important thing to note: the specialist will usually produce a report containing recommendations for a child's individual education plan. Having invited the specialist in to give them guidance, the school must be prepared to follow that advice. Usually all the provisions available at Stage 2 are still appropriate but they will be offered at a more intense level. Children will be offered more time with a specialist teacher, the SENCO will spend more time advising the teacher and so on.

Kind of provision	Example
Increased small group teaching from a designated special needs teacher. The specialist will almost certainly recommend the kinds of programme covered in Chapters 2–6.	As at Stage 2. Actual amounts of time will vary from school to school and from child to child.
Increased regular support from another teacher in the mainstream classroom.	At secondary school the aim will be to increase the range of subjects in which a support teacher can be present.

Kind of provision	Example
Increased support from a non-teaching assistant in the mainstream classroom.	Many schools are exploring the possibility of using LSAs for this kind of support. Often a fully qualified teacher is not necessary for the tasks which are required.
Assessment and monitoring by the specialist and SENCO.	Ideally the specialist will be able to attend each review meeting and give advice and guidance on the SENCO's report on the child's progress following the recommendations made by the specialist.
More curriculum materials adapted by or under the guidance of the SENCO.	For the child at Stage 3 it may be necessary for the SENCO to become more involved in helping class and subject teachers adapt the materials they use with dyslexic children in their classes. This cannot all be done at once. Most schools are gradually building up their stock of adapted material.
More frequent help for children with concepts and skills which they will be encountering in future lessons.	The specialist may well have given advice in this area on the best approaches to use with a child. If the child has been seen by an educational psychologist then there may be clues in the his or her learning profile which will give an insight. The child may be a strong visual learner. This will mean that new concepts would be better explained using visual cues and diagrams.
Increased advice on programmes, materials and methods from a specialist teacher. Programmes for class devised by the SENCO or special needs teacher.	Again the specialist's report should assist here. It is likely to recommend structured, cumulative, thorough and multi-sensory programmes.

Stage 5:   Children with severe difficulties

We have not forgotten Stage 4. This is when statutory assessment takes place. It is a kind of limbo period for the child when the school will continue to make provision. The table lists the wide range of forms of support which can be provided by a statement. It is important to emphasise that the school's responsibility for meeting a child's special needs does not end when a statement is agreed for a child. Unless the child is placed in full-time special provision the school still has a responsibility to meet the child's needs in conjunction with the Authority. In other words, in most cases, if the child stays in the same school, then the support offered by that school at Stage 3 should continue. The statemented provision is in addition to the extra funded by the Authority.

Kind of provision	Comment
Small group support for direct teaching by a specialist teacher in their local school or specialist centre.	We would argue that specialist teachers for statemented dyslexic children should hold a specific special needs qualification. Ideally they will have a qualification to teach dyslexic children which has been recognised by the British Dyslexia Association. There is one caveat: an effective teacher without a qualification is better than an ineffective one with one. How much time is allocated will vary from child to child and LEA to LEA. A minimum of one hour a week up to a maximum of five covers the usual range. It is difficult to advise parents or teachers here; so much depends on the individual child. There are other factors too. One hour a week of individual tuition may be as beneficial as two hours with in a group of three or four or vice versa. If you are unsure seek advice.
Resourced mainstream school	Many authorities are seeking to establish this kind of facility for their dyslexic pupils who do not make sufficient progress with small group support in their local school or specialist centre. The resourced school will offer a mix of intensive individual or small group specialist tuition, informed support within mainstream lessons and mainstream teachers who are familiar with the needs of dyslexic pupils. The main advantage of these resourced facilities is that it allows able dyslexic children to follow the mainstream curriculum appropriate to their age and ability. Without them the alternative could be either special classes or special school.
Special class or unit	The nature of these classes vary. Some are full-time, some are part-time. Some are exclusively for dyslexic children, some also cater for children with more general learning difficulties. In essence what they will offer is an alternative curriculum. For this reason, they are probably more appropriate for dyslexic children of lower ability who have difficulties understanding the curriculum offered to their peers in the mainstream class.
Special schools	A few LEAs maintain specialist schools for dyslexic pupils. The quality of education they offer is usually very high but we do not believe it appropriate for dyslexic children to be forced to leave mainstream education. The emphasis should be placed on resourcing mainstream schools to meet the needs of dyslexic children. By definition children with *specific* learning difficulties should be able to follow the mainstream *general* curriculum if they are correctly taught and supported. We can see a case for very severely dyslexic children whose learning difficulties are so compounded by other factors that they cannot emotionally cope with mainstream education possible needing such provision. However, these children are very, very rare indeed.
Specialist independent schools for dyslexic children	See previous item.

Conclusion

We have tried to cover the whole continuum of provision available for dyslexic pupils in this brief chapter. However, in an educational system as diverse as our own, there will be many other examples of different forms of assistance for them. The main test of any provision is its effectiveness. We have known some children to attend specialist independent schools and not make adequate progress. We have known others who have attended their local school to be taught for 2 hours a week by an exceptional special needs teacher and class teacher and they have blossomed. The main consideration here is that the provision which is offered to children should be regularly reviewed and evaluated. The targets set at Stages 2 to 5 are vital to this. They are not pretty words designed to make it look as though something is happening. They are the yardstick against which the effectiveness of a child's educational plan should be measured.

If the targets are consistently not reached, then they are either too hard or the teaching programme needs to be reconsidered. Both possibilities should be carefully considered at each review meeting. If they are consistently reached quickly then either they are too easy or the teaching programme is working well for that child. It is important to establish which is the case.

A major obstacle to the progress of all children with special needs, and especially dyslexic children, is the low expectations that teachers and parents sometimes hold for them. If you treat children as slow and unintelligent, they will behave slowly and dully. Treat them as able pupils, capable of rapid progress, and they are far more likely to progress.

Finally, the most important contributors to children's special needs provision are the children themselves and their parents. If the children are well motivated, confident and happy they are far more likely to learn and progress. They are far more likely to be well motivated and confident if they have their parent's full backing, time and encouragement.

Summary of Chapter 10

This chapter:

- showed how the extent of children's special educational needs should be matched by the extent of the provision to meet those needs;

- described how matching extent of need to extent of provision relates to dyslexic children;

- illustrated what kind of provision is usually made available for dyslexic children at Stages 1, 2, 3 and 5 of the UK Code of Practice for Children with Special Educational Needs.

A Final Word

The Green Paper for children with special educational needs

At the time of publication, a Green Paper had been issued in England and Wales which, if confirmed in resultant legislation, would have major implications for dyslexic children. A Green Paper is a consultation document. It signals an intention by the Government to change the law in the ways the Paper specifies. Following consultation, a White Paper is written. This White Paper will then proceed through the Parliamentary processes until, if successful, it emerges as new legislation. The Green Papers in England and Wales differed from each other, but each shared a number of significant recommendations for dyslexic children. On the whole we welcome both Green Papers for dyslexic children. They contain a number of sensible and innovatory ideas, which should improve identification of, and provision for, these children. These are also listed, along with their potential implications for dyslexic children. We cannot find a major fault with any of them. Taken together they offer a sensible and practical step forward.

The Green Paper for Special Educational Needs in England and Wales

Recommendation	Implication for dyslexic children
Children with special educational needs should be identified earlier	This must be good for dyslexic children. Early identification is vital if their progress is to be maximised. In line with this recommendation, all English and Welsh schools must in future assess their reception age children on a new Baseline Assessment Test. The results of this assessment should also help to identify potential dyslexic pupils. If so, then there is another crucial step: any needs that are identified must also be properly met. Extra resourcing must be found and channeled into these children whose needs are identified earlier.
Expectations of children with special educational needs will be higher	If expectations are raised then this should be a very positive move forward for dyslexic children. Their potential can so easily be underestimated. For instance, the content of their writing may be excellent, but because it looks untidy or the spelling is poor, it can receive lower marks than it actually deserves. Dyslexic children should be set high targets of achievement and have their real achievements acknowledged by their teachers.

Recommendation	*Implication for dyslexic children*
There will be increased use of Information Communication Technology (ICT)	Throughout this book we have stressed the importance, the growing importance, of ICT for dyslexic children. There is huge potential for technology to help them show what they know in alternative ways to writing, or in assisting their writing (see Chapter 7).
All children being assessed towards a statement of special need should be given the support of an independent Named Person	The Green Paper recommends that the independent Named Person should be agreed with parents at the start, not the end, of the assessment process. This must be a helpful improvement for parents who require this kind of informed source of support and information (see Chapter 9).
Parents and LEAs should seek reconciliation on the contents of statements which are in dispute, rather than go immediately to Tribunal	Anything which produces an acceptable compromise to both parties, must be better than the long-drawn out appeal process (see Chapter 9).
The Code of Practice for Special Educational Needs should be revised to reduce paperwork and bureaucracy	Anything which concentrates teachers' and parents' time on actually teaching and helping children, rather than writing about teaching and helping them, must be welcomed (see Chapter 8).
The number of statements issued by many LEAs should be reduced. The Green Paper envisages a system whereby the Stage 3 Individual Education Plan (8.6) is strengthened, so that there is less need to move towards a statement: under this system, provision formerly only available through a statement, can be made at Stage 3	The main British dyslexic associations have reacted with some hostility to this proposal. They fear that children will lose the legally guaranteed access to extra support which a statement can provide. We do not take this view. The statementing process is lengthy, expensive and bureaucratic. If a suitable Stage 3 process can be devised, which will ensure that children receive the support they need, for the time they need it, then this must be preferable to the inevitable requirement to move to statutory assessment. We would recommend that only children who do not make sufficient progress with the extra provision they receive, via a strengthened Stage 3 Individual Plan, should be considered for a statement.
The Green Paper recommends that more children with special educational needs should be included in mainstream schools	We have a simple perspective on this. We do not believe any dyslexic child, whose difficulties are restricted to dyslexia, should be in a special school. By definition, they are capable of understanding and following the mainstream curriculum. They should be given increased support to access the mainstream curriculum, not placed in a special schools because they have difficulty in doing so (see Chapter 10).

Recommendation	*Implication for dyslexic children*
There should be improved training for all professionals involved in teaching or supporting children with special educational needs, including extra training for student teachers, newly qualified teachers and non-teaching assistants	This is a very positive move for dyslexic children. Awareness of their specific educational needs has been growing for many years, but it is still rather piecemeal. Increased training is especially needed for training teachers, class teachers and managers. More specialist dyslexia-trained teachers are also required.
Educational psychologists need to have their roles widened so that they may be more effective (Chapter 8)	This also relates to the need or not for dyslexic children to have statements. If a child is to have a statement, then an educational psychologist must give that child an in-depth assessment and follow this up with advice in the form of a detailed assessment report. The value of these reports should not be underestimated, but sometimes the psychologist's time might be more profitably spent actually working with children and their teachers, on improving the quality of the programmes of study they are following in class.
Responsibilities for speech therapy and other therapies should be clarified	Dyslexic children often have related speech and language difficulties or fine motor difficulties, which require the intervention of a specialist therapist. The current law says that if a particular therapy is specified in Part 3 of a child's statement, then the Health Authority has the prime responsibility for providing that therapy. However, if they cannot offer it, then the LEA must. This Alice in Wonderland situation has caused much friction between Health Trusts and LEAs for many years. It has sometimes prevented children from receiving the therapy they deserve. If the law in this area is tightened up and clarified, many children will have been done a great service.
The transition of children from school to post-school needs improving. Examples of good practice in this area will be collected to improve general practice	In many schools and LEAs, this area of practice must be improved. Dyslexic children may well be missing out on their life chances, because they are ill-informed at vital points in their careers. They especially need expert and informed advice on careers and further or higher education. Currently, children with statements are entitled to have a Transition Plan written for them. This Plan will help all agencies involved with them to plan post school opportunities together. However, actual practice in this appears to be rather patchy. If statements are not to be maintained for as many dyslexic children as they are now, then consideration should be given to extending the best Transition Plan practice to all children at Stage 3 (see Chapter 9).

Recommendation	*Implication for dyslexic children*
Teaching staff will have improved skills in dealing with children with behavioural difficulties	There is an increasing recognition that dyslexic children are more likely than some other children to experience emotional and behavioural difficulties. While we would argue that these difficulties should reduce or disappear if their learning difficulties have been met, it must be to the advantage of all children if teachers do strengthen their skills of behaviour management

Meeting Special Educational Needs – A Programme of Action

Literally as this this book was going to publication the Government (UK) issued its response to consultation on the green paper, called *Meeting Special Educational Needs – A Programme of Action*. In the following table we have identified where this programme is different from or adds to what we have just written about the Green Paper. We have concentrated only on those things which may affect children with dyslexia. (The Welsh Paper was not issued at the time of publication. It will probably have small but significant variations to the English version.)

Area	*Action Plan Recommendation*	*Date*
Early Identification	All children in the first half term of their reception year in school are given a baseline assessment. This assessment will establish their skills and knowledge when they first begin statutory education. This assessment will help schools identify children with potential dyslexic problems. It will for instance allow an at-a-glance opportunity for teachers to see which children have the kind of uneven profile which could indicate a potential dyslexic problem. Children might show themselves, for example, to be well above average in creative or scientific skills but well behind in simple writing or reading skills. As information from Baseline assessment grows we believe it could develop into a reliable means of identifying children with dyslexic type difficulties and thus to intervene early to stop those difficulties becoming more pronounced.	1998
Revising the Code of Practice	The Code of Practice will be revised. The main changes proposed: 1. To reduce the paperwork involved in writing Individual Education Plans (IEPs) it is recommended that each child has three or four priority targets set for key areas of skill. 2. To remove the current Stage 1, restricting the Code to children who need help which is additional to or different from that which is available for all children.	2000/1

Area	Action Plan Recommendation	Date
	3. To define help for children as either being available from school – *school support* – or from the LEA – *support plus*. This will replace the need for the previously proposed strengthened Stage 3 contract instead of a statement. Parents did not want to lose the guarantee of support brought by a statement.	1999
	4. Improve the quantity and quality of school support by increasing the funding made available to meet children's needs at the school based stages of the Code.	1999
Statements	1. The Green Paper's specific reference to most dyslexic children not requiring statements is omitted. Instead the Action Plan says that over time they expect 'the special educational needs of most children who do not have severe, long term or lifelong complex medical or physical needs will be met without a statement.'	2000/1
	2. Each child's statement should include outcomes or targets whose achievement will show that a statement is no longer necessary. Subsequent annual reviews for that child should carefully consider the continuing need for a statement by seeing if the outcomes have been achieved.	
	3. Transition reviews should take place in Year 9. They will be co-ordinated by schools not LEAs.	
	4. There will be timescales laying down how quickly LEAs should respond to SEN Tribunal judgements.	
LEAs	1. LEAs will be required to publish information about what schools should normally provide for children with special educational needs from their budgets.	1999
	2. Our reading of the new 'Fair Funding' arrangements for schools is that LEAs will continue to be allowed to directly fund extra support for the most severely dyslexic children, rather than this funding being added to schools' budgets.	
Training issues	1. All training teachers will be taught how to identify children with special educational needs and how to provide for those needs in their own classes.	1998
	2. The Government is consulting on establishing standards for specialist teachers, such as teachers of dyslexic children. These standards will then be published.	Not stated
Parents	1. All LEAs must have a parent partnership scheme to provide parents with independent information about SEN procedures, school based provision and other support.	1999
	2. Parents of children with SEN will also be entitled to access to an independent parental supporter.	1999
	3. LEAs will be expected to establish conciliation arrangements, with an independent element, for resolving disputes with parents.	2000

Area	*Action Plan Recommendation*	*Date*
Finally, the child . . .	LEAs and schools will be required to have regard to the wishes and feelings of children when making decisions about meeting their SEN.	2000/1

The Way Forward

The aim of this book has been to give parents and teachers a broad overview of dyslexia and show them how they can help if their children or their pupils are dyslexic. We have tried to give positive and practical guidance in understanding what it means to be dyslexic. This has meant that at times we have had to stress the difficulties associated with dyslexia, the stresses and strains that it can impose on children who are attempting to show their potential in the demanding climate of modern schools. We want to leave you on a more upbeat note, by reassuring you that being dyslexic is not a catastrophe.

We accept that dyslexia can never be fully cured but its negative effects can be greatly reduced with the right kind of intervention and support. With appropriate teaching, high motivation and increased self-confidence, improvements in performance can be dramatic and long lasting. As you will see, we firmly believe that the need to acquire the basic skills of reading, writing and arithmetic will become increasingly less important as more and more technological advances make them redundant. However, we would not wish to suggest that children's ability to read and independently of machines will become unimportant. This may never be true. There is something special and private about being able to lose yourself in world of the printed page or to generate your own thoughts with just a pen and paper. All children, including dyslexic children, will continue to value these skills and experiences. All children are entitled to be able to read, write and calculate independently. But for dyslexic children to succeed at school across the curriculum, and for dyslexic employees to compete on an equal playing field with their colleagues at work, the new technology is vital.

Twenty years ago, to be labelled dyslexic meant that others might see you as unintelligent or 'backward'. Thanks to the work of many pioneers across the world, we have now come to a time which could be called the 'renaissance' of dyslexia. Being dyslexic in the next millennium will be seen as a positive advantage. Being a bright, dyslexic pupil or employee will open doors once firmly slammed shut. We believe that there will be positive discrimination amongst schools for dyslexic pupils and amongst employers towards dyslexic employees, as they are sought for their unique and valued thinking skills.

The key to this development is scientific advance. Constant, dynamic improvement in the field of information technology will free dyslexic people from the fetters imposed on them by their poor mechanical skills of literacy and numeracy. In the future machines will read for us. Computers will spell for us. Computers will write for us. Computers will calculate for us. These simple, unobtrusive machines will reduce the acquisition of literacy and numeracy to an ability to push the right buttons at the right time. When these machines become commonplace, those people with poor mechanical skills but divergent and creative styles of thinking, who have something different and innovative to say, will be empowered. They will rise above their more literate and numerate peers who have formerly prospered. They will rise above those who so easily rise to the top of the class today, with their workmanlike but finely honed skills of ever precise spelling and ever accurate calculation. So the future looks bright for dyslexic children and adults. We are poised on the threshold of a new era for them. In this bright new world, dyslexic people will continue to lead the way in innovation and thought, as did the dyslexic Michaelangelo. They will become respected members of a society which recognises and values their worth. In that spirit we will end with the following advice for dyslexic children of today:

DYSLEXIA DOES RULE, OK!

- Believe in yourself;

- Use the new technology to show what you know;

- Use your dyslexic strengths to your advantage;

- Work hard;

- Set yourself realistic short- and long-term targets;

- Do not give up – a struggle often comes before success;

- Nothing succeeds like success;

- If you are working hard at school and you are not learning, then you need to be taught differently;

- Be happy, the future is yours.

Glossary of Terms, Phrases and Acronyms Used in This Book

Access to the curriculum	The importance of this phrase is that it refers to making the curriculum accessible to the child, not the child to the curriculum.
AMBDA	Associate Member of the British Dyslexia Association.
Annual General Meeting	The Governing Body of every UK maintained school must hold an open Annual General Meeting for all parents of the school, to discuss the Annual Report on the school issued earlier. Implementation of the School's SEN Policy must be reported on at this meeting.
Annual Review	An Annual Review (UK) should be conducted on every child's statement on or before the anniversary of the last statement or annual review.
Apprentice reading	A method in which the child learns to read by practice with, and support from, a more accomplished reader.
Appendices	Formal name for the reports prepared for a statement assessment.
Ascenders	Letters which have upright tails: b, d, f, h, k, l, t.
Assisted reading	Methods of teaching reading which match the learning reader with a more accomplished reader. See also apprentice reading, paired reading and peer tutoring.
ATSBDA	Approved Teacher Status of the British Dyslexia Association.
Auditory memory	The ability to remember what you hear.
Auditory perception	How accurately children hear information: this usually refers to their ability to correctly hear the sounds made by words, letters and numbers.
Auditory rehearsal	A technique which can be taught to children of saying a word slowly to themselves, usually aloud, as an aid to remembering and recalling its spelling.
Auditory sequential memory	The ability to remember sequences that have been heard, i.e. the order of letters in a word.
Automatic memory	Those things which have been remembered so well that they can be instantly recalled.
BDA	British Dyslexia Association (see useful addresses). An independent organisation which promotes the interests of dyslexics.

Befriender	Someone who will support parents in their negotiations with schools and LEAs, on educational matters concerning their children.
Breve	Short vowel sound. e.g. the sound of *a* in *cat* or *e* in *bet*.
Calligraphy	The art of handwriting.
CD-ROM	Compact Disc- Read Only Memory, i.e. you can only read information from the CD, you cannot change or add to it.
Chunking	This is the technique, when writing, of grouping words together in their natural chunks or syllables and then combining them into continuous text, building the chunks up. The technique can also be used to help children remember information such as telephone numbers and work with syllables.
Closed letters	In cursive writing, closed letters are those which should be closed over, e.g. *a, d, o*.
Code of Practice for the Assessment and Identification of Special Educational Needs	In the UK, this Code provides a mixture of guidance and instruction to schools and LEAs on the procedures they should follow, and the responsibilities they must fulfil, in meeting children's special educational needs.
Cognitive ability	This refers to children's ability to think and reason.
Compound words	Words made of complete words joined together, e.g. *woodwork, classroom, headboard*.
Consonant	A letter which is not a vowel: *b, c, d, f, g, h, j, k, l, m, n, o, p, q, r, s, t, v, w, x, (y), z*.
Consonant blends	Two or more consonants blended together to make a single sound, in which the individual sounds can still be heard, e.g. *st, bl, gr, str*.
Consonant digraphs	When two or more consonants together make a different sound to that of their individual sounds, e.g. *ch, sh, th, ph*.
Cross-laterality	Most of us are naturally either left-sided or right-sided, e.g. some people naturally prefer to use their left eye, left hand and left foot. Some people are cross-lateral; they may be left-eyed but right-handed, or left-footed and right-eared.
Cross-curricular skill	A skill which is needed across most or all subjects in the curriculum, e.g. reading, speaking, listening.
Cursive writing	Joined-up handwriting.
Decoding	Breaking words down into their individual sounds.
Descenders	Letters which have hanging tails: *f, g, j, p, q, y*.
DfE	The Department for Education (UK).

Differentiation	The individual delivery of the curriculum, to make it more accessible for children with SEN.
Digraph	Two or more letters making one sound, e.g. *ai, sh, sph*.
Diphthong	Two vowels next to one another whose sounds glide together, e.g. *ow* in *cow*, *ou* in *out* or *oy* in *toy*.
Directionality	The direction in which something should go, such as calculating from left to right or the correct orientation of a letter.
Disapplication of the National Curriculum	A child's entitlement to the full National Curriculum may be disapplied on a temporary basis or permanent basis. A temporary disapplication may be up to a maximum of 12 months. A permanent disapplication is only available through a child's statement.
Double consonant	e.g. *bl, tr, sh, pl*.
Dyscalculia	Specific difficulties with number.
Dyseidetic	A weakness in remembering whole word shapes and a poor memory for letters.
Dysgraphia	Specific difficulty with handwriting.
Dyslexia Institute	An independent UK organisation which promotes the interests of dyslexics. It also offers teaching support although charges are made for this. See Useful Addresses.
Dysphonetic	A weakness in being able to perceive words by their sounds, or sound out words phonically.
Educational Psychologist	An expert in the UK in the way children learn and behave. He or she must have taught, have a psychology degree (or equivalent) and have a further degree in educational psychology.
ESW	Educational Social Worker; sometimes known as Educational Welfare Officers (UK).
Encoding	Building words up from their individual sounds.
Exam dispensation	In the UK, dyslexic children can be given help to allow them to show what they know in their final compulsory school examinations, GCSE (e.g. extra time) to complete an examination. This makes the exam system fairer for them.
Expressive language	The ability to communicate thoughts and feelings in speech and gesture.
Fast-track referrals	Procedure which allows children with sudden and severe needs to miss out some of the early assessment stages (UK).
Feint	The width between lines.

Final statement	The final statement is issued after any negotiations between parents and the LEA have ended – with or without agreement. Parents have a right of appeal to the SEN Tribunal against the contents of a statement (UK).
Fine motor skills	Small movements of the body, typically finger and hand movements, like drawing, handwriting or tying laces.
Five SEN stages	The Code of Practice (UK) recommends that children's SEN are identified and met at one of five stages, on a continuum from Stage 1, least severe, to Stage 5, most severe, difficulties.
Further Education or FE Colleges	FE is a UK term describing post-school education. It is distinct from Higher Education, which specifically refers to institutions which offer degree and postgraduate courses.
Funding Council	The central body which administers funding for grant-maintained schools (UK).
GCSE	General Certificate of Education. State examination in the UK administered at the end of Key Stage 4.
General Practitioner or GP	UK term for a non-specialist doctor who serves the local community.
GNVQ	General National Vocational Qualification (UK).
Grant-maintained school	A UK term describing a state school funded centrally rather than by the local council. Soon to be superseded by Foundation Schools.
Gross motor skills	Large movements of the limbs and body, like running, hopping, throwing and catching.
HAG	Handwriting Action Grid.
Hand-eye coordination	How well the brain gets the hand to do what the eye is telling it to do.
Hardware	Technological machines, especially computers.
Hear to write	You hear the word and write it.
High-frequency words	Words which occur most often in written English.
Higher Education Colleges	Universities and colleges which offer degree and postgraduate courses. See also 'Further Education'.
Homophones	Words with the same sounds but different meanings and spellings, e.g. *sail, sale* or *meat, meet*.
ICT	Information Communication Technology.
IEP	Individual Education Plan.
Inclusion	The right of all children to be educated within ordinary schools.
Independent school	In the UK, this is a school which is funded by parental fees.

Infant school/class	UK description for school or class for children aged 5–7.
Integration	Being educated within the ordinary school or classroom.
Intuitive Colorometer	A device which measures children's visual perception. Similar to Scotopic Sensitivity Syndrome.
Irlen Syndrome	See 'Scotopic Sensitivity Syndrome'.
IQ	Intelligence Quotient.
Junior school/class	UK description for school or class for children aged 7–11.
Key Words	Refers to the McNally/Murray Key Words which represent the 200 most commonly encountered words in written English (see also 'sight words').
Kinaesthetic	Sense of movement, feel and touch.
KS1	UK Key Stage 1, Years 1 and 2 (typically aged 5 to 7).
KS2	UK Key Stage 2, Years 3 to 6 (typically aged 7 to 11).
KS3	UK Key Stage 3, Years 7 to 9 (typically aged 11 to 14).
KS4	UK Key Stage 4, Years 10 and 11 (typically aged 14 to 16).
Learning Support Teacher	In the UK, a general term for teachers who specialise in offering support for children with special educational needs.
LEA/Local Education Authority	In the UK, aspects of the administration of education are managed by Local Education Authorities (LEAs) which are in turn run by local councils. The power of LEAs has significantly diminished over the last decade with more and more decision making and funding delegated to schools.
Lexicon	A personal bank of words which can be read or written.
Linguist	A specialist in the study of language.
LMS	Local Management of Schools: a UK term for the process where the budget is delegated to the Governing Body of maintained schools to manage.
LMSS	Local Management of Special Schools: a UK term for the process where the budget is delegated to the Governing Body of maintained special schools to manage.
Look and Say	Reading method which emphasises whole word learning.
Long vowel sound	The vowel makes the same sound as its name, e.g. *a* as in *cake*, *i* as in *bite*.
Lower case writing	Not capital letters.
Macron	Symbol for long vowel sound.
Maintained school	A school funded through local and national taxation.

Mainstream school/class	Ordinary school or class (i.e. not a special school or class).
Mind maps	A visual way of structuring thoughts and plans on paper.
Mirror words	Words which have been read or spelt the wrong way round, like *saw* for *was*.
Mnemonic	An aid to memory. The first letters of a striking phrase are used to trigger the memory: e.g. **R**O**Y** **G**et **B**ack **I**n **T**he **V**an for the colours of the rainbow: red, orange, yellow, green, blue, indigo and violet.
Multi-sensory techniques	Methods of teaching which encourage children to learn using more than one sense: 'seeing as they feel as they say as they write'.
Named Officer	The LEA Officer who is the first point of contact for parents during and after the statementing process (UK).
Named Person	Someone who will give support and information to parents whose children are being assessed towards a possible statement of special educational need (UK).
National Curriculum/NC	UK National Curriculum: *Key Stages 1 and 2*: Primary: English, Mathematics, Science, Information Technology, History, Geography, Music, Art, PE, + Welsh in Wales. *Key Stages 3 and 4*: + Modern Foreign Language
Non-verbal	Without words. For example, using signs and gestures rather than words.
Note-in-Lieu	This is a note in lieu of a statement (UK). As its name suggests it is written at the end of the assessment process, when a statement is not considered necessary.
NTA	Non-teaching assistant (UK). Also known as Learning Support Assistants (LSAs), Special School Assistants (SSAs), Nursery Nurses (NNEBs), Project Workers and Ancillary Support Workers (ASWs).
Nursery school/ class	UK description for school or class for children below compulsory school age of five years.
One-to-one tuition or 1:1	This does not always mean one child and one teacher. It can refer to a child being part of a small group where the attention which each child receives is always one to one, but is not constant.
Onset	The initial consonant in words, e.g. the *m* in *mat*.
Open letters	Letters which should not be closed over, e.g. *h, u, w*.
Orientation	Getting it the right way round; being sure of the correct direction, e.g. not writing *was* for *saw*, *b* for *d*.
Orthography	Spelling according to everyday usage.

Overlearning	This refers to the need for some children to be given many opportunities to learn the same information or skill in a series of different settings; to fix it firmly in their memory.
Paired reading	A method of learning to read in which the learner reads simultaneously with a more able reader. Gradually the better reader drops out and the learner becomes more and more independent.
Peer group	Children of the same age.
Peer tutoring	Children being supported in their learning by other children.
Pen/pencil grip	The correct way to hold the pen or pencil for writing. The grip is different for right and left handers.
Performance Indicators	In the UK, Local Education Authorities must publish key performance data to show they are offering an effective service. The number of proposed statements issued in 18 weeks is one indicator.
Perseverance	Usually this means the ability to keep going when the odds are against you. In reading and writing , however, it can also mean adding extra letters to a word, e.g. *rememberer*.
Phoneme	A single sound, e.g. *b, ch, str*.
Phonics	A reading method which emphasises building up and breaking down words, according to their individual sounds.
Prefix	A word beginning, e.g. *pre, id, un* which changes the meaning of the word when added to it; e.g. *like* becomes its opposite with *dis*: *dislike*.
Primary school	UK description for school or class for children aged 5–11.
Proposed Statement	A draft form of statement sent to parents to consider (UK).
Psycholinguistic reading method	Reading method which emphasises learning to read by reading stimulating and interesting texts.
Public school	In the UK, private, i.e. not state-funded funded schools, are known as public schools. They are also known as private schools and non-maintained schools.
Quartiles	The four quartiles of the alphabet: *a–d, e–l, m–r*, and *s–z*.
Quotient	A quotient is a useful way of showing children's scores on a test compared to the average. Average scores usually lie between 85 and 115 with a mean of 100.
Reading accuracy age	A measure of how accurately children read.
Reading comprehension age	A measure of how well children understand what they read.

Reading cues	Clues or cues which assist the reader to tackle new or difficult words, e.g. the context of a word or its initial letter sound may help the reader to read it.
Reading fluency age	A measure of the speed at which children read.
Reading scheme books	Books which have been written to help children learn to read. They have usually been graded for difficulty.
Real books	Books which do not belong to reading schemes: literature, handbooks, football programmes. Books which are written to be read as against being written to help children learn to read.
Recall of digits test	This test assesses short term auditory memory.
Reception class	A UK description for the school year before Year 1.
Receptive language ability	The ability to understand what is said to you.
Reinforcement	This refers to two things: 1. the need to reinforce children's good progress or behaviour by emphasising it with recognition or reward. 2. the need to emphasise or force home newly acquired knowledge and skills by reinforcing it with revision and overlearning.
Reversals	Letters, words, parts of word and numbers which have been read or written the wrong way round. e.g. *kool* for *look, q* for *p*.
Rime	The final vowel and consonant in a word, e.g. *at* in *mat*.
Roots of words	The core part of a word, e.g. *act* in *react, gram* in *telegram*. The root contains the word's core meaning.
SALT	Speech and Language Therapist.
SATS	Standard Assessment Tests/Tasks: end of Key Stage national tests undertaken by all pupils in England and Wales.
Scanning	A technique, which can be taught to children, for quickly extracting the essential information from a text without reading every word, most useful when looking for particular piece of information in a reference book.
Scotopic Sensitivity Syndrome	Children identified as having this syndrome tend to have a difficulty with visual perception. This difficulty is often in the form of the child being unusually sensitive to certain wave lengths of light. Also known as Irlen Syndrome.
See to write	You see the word and write it.
Secondary school/class	UK description for school or class for children aged 11 and over.

Self-esteem	How well individual value themselves and have a positive image of themselves. Related to concepts of self-image. It is generally thought that the more positive a child's self-image and self-esteem is as a learner, the more effectively he or she will learn.
Semantic	Related to the meaning of words.
SEN	Special Educational Needs.
SEN Policy	In the UK every maintained school must have a Special Needs Policy, available to parents and reported on annually to parents.
SEN Register	Every maintained school must maintain a register of all children who have SEN (UK).
SEN Tribunal	Formal body which arbitrates between parents and LEAs on the contents of final statements (UK).
Short-term auditory memory	The ability to remember what you have just heard.
Short-term visual memory	The ability to remember what you have just seen.
Short vowel	The sound of *a* in *cat*, *e* in *bet*, *i* in *hit*, *o* in *cot* and *u* in *cut*.
Silent letters	Letters which do not appear to have a sound of their own in some words such as the *k* in *know*, the *h* in *ghost* or the *g* in *gnat*.
Sixth Form College/School	UK description for school or class for Years 11–13 (aged 16–19).
Software	Computer programs.
Sound-symbol correspondence	The link between a letter(s) and its sound(s). Another, related phrase is 'sound–symbol matching'.
Spacing	When the child is handwriting, this refers to the spaces between letters and words.
Spatial awareness	Awareness of figures in relation to each other and the space around them.
Special Educational Needs Coordinator (SENCO)	The teacher responsible for co-ordinating the day to day implementation of each school's Special Needs Policy.
Special arrangements	In the UK special arrangements can be made to allow children with special educational needs to show what they know in the Key Stage Tests. Special Arrangements range from having the test read to them to having someone write answers for them. The SENCO should organise this.
SpLD (Dyslexia)	Specific Learning Difficulties (Dyslexia), the most widely recognised name for the condition in the UK.

Specialist teachers	In this book this term refers to teachers who have acquired extra qualifications and experience in teaching children with special educational needs.
Spell-checker	A hand held device, the size and shape of a calculator, used to help children quickly check their spellings. Most word processing programmes also possess an internal spell-checker.
Spiky profile	This term is used when children's performance on a test of general ability is uneven. When this occurs it will give an uneven or spiky test profile, which is often taken to indicate that the children have a dyslexic type difficulty.
Standardised Test	A test which has been established by trialling it with a large number (usually 1000+) of pupils. A standardised test score allows comparisons between the results achieved by a child on the test and an estimated average score for his or her age. For instance, reading ages and quotients are usually gained from tests which have been standardised.
Statement	A legal document which confirms child has special Educational needs over and above that which an ordinary school could be expected to provide. It identifies child's needs and provision and placement to meet those needs (UK).
Statutory assessment	The official term for the assessment process which may lead to a statement of special educational need (UK).
Study skills	Those skills which will enhance a child's ability to learn, remember and reproduce information, concepts and skills.
Suffix	A word ending, e.g. *tion, ing, er*.
Syntactic	How words are put together in phrases, sentences and paragraphs.
Tasks	A UK term: some children, including dyslexic children do not readily show what they know on written tests. Tasks, or activity-based tests, are provided for these pupils. Task assessments have equal status with ordinary short tests in UK National Assessments.
Teacher Assessments/TAs	This is a UK term: as well as their pupils taking SATs, teachers make their own assessments of their National Curriculum levels at the end of Key Stages. These are called Teacher Assessments or TAs.
Telescoping words	Shortening the spelling of words, e.g. *rember* for *remember*.
Thesaurus	A book which groups words according to their meanings. It is useful for looking up alternative words with the same or similar meanings. Most word-processing programmes and spell-checkers have an in-built thesaurus.
Transition Plan	A form of Annual Review for children over the age of fourteen who have statements. The Plan aims to assist and inform the child's transition to post-school life (UK).

Triple consonant	e.g. *str, spr, scr*.
Underachiever	A child who is not performing to his or her full ability. For a dyslexic child, this would often refer to their skills in literacy/numeracy not reflecting the potential shown by their achievement in other areas.
Upper case writing	Capital letters.
Verbal	In words.
Visual discrimination	The ability to visually distinguish one thing from another, e.g. *were* from *where* or *how* from *who*.
Visual memory	The ability to remember what you have seen.
Visual perception	This describes how accurately children see information. This usually refers to their ability to correctly see the shapes made by words, letters and numbers.
Visual pegs	Visual aids to a child's memory, such as helping them to associate a picture of letter with its sound, e.g. a picture of a dog for *d*.
Visual recall	Recalling information visually, e.g. recalling the correct sequence of letters in a word.
Visual sequential memory	The ability to remember the sequence of what you have seen, e.g. remembering the order of letters in a word.
Vowel	A letter which is not a consonant: *a, e, i, o, u, (y)*.
Vowel digraphs	This is when two letters together make a vowel sound which is different to their individual sounds in sequence, e.g. *ea, ai, ei, aw, ay*.
Word-finding difficulty	The difficulty children have in recalling words, which are in their vocabulary, when they are needed.
Word-reading test	This kind of test measures children's ability to read single words in isolation.

Books and Resources

Very many books have been published on dyslexia. Our booklist is minute in comparison. We have restricted our list to books we have personally used and found helpful. We have eliminated very technical or very 'academic' books. Those books marked with * are probably more suitable to readers who wish to acquire a more in-depth knowledge of the subject.

General Reading on Dyslexia

Augur, J. *Information on Dyslexia for Schools*, British Dyslexia Association.
Augur, J. *This Book Doesn't Make Sense – A Practical Guide for Parents for Helping the Dyslexic Child*, Amethyst Books.
Augur, J. *Games and Activities for Parents and Children to Play*, British Dyslexia Association.
Beugin, M. *Attention Deficit Disorder: A Guide for Parents and Teachers*, Detselig Enterprises.
Blight, J. *Practical Guide to Dyslexia*, Egon.
British Dyslexia Association (Jane Jacobsen ed.), *The Dyslexia Handbook 1998*. (This is a must, practical and packed with information. You have to join the BDA to receive it.)
Buzan, A. *The Mind Map Book: Radiant Thinking*, BBC Books
Davis, R. *The Gift of Dyslexia*, Souvenir Press.
Heaton, P. *Dyslexic Parents in Need*, Whurr.
* Miles, T.R. *Dyslexia, the Pattern of Difficulties*, Whurr.
Miles, T.R. and Miles, E. *Help for Dyslexic Children*, Routledge.
Miles, T.R. and Gilroy, D.E. *Dyslexia at College*, Routledge.
Miles, T.R. and Varma, V.P. (eds) *Dyslexia and Stress*, Whurr.
Ott, P. *How to Detect and Manage Dyslexia*, Heinemann.
Pollock, J. and Waller, E. *Day to Day Dyslexia in the Classroom*, Routledge.
Portswood, M. *Developmental Dyspraxia*, Durham County Council.
* Pumfrey, P. and Reason, R. *Specific Learning Difficulties (Dyslexia), Challenges and Responses*, Routledge.
Riddick, B. *Living with Dyslexia*, Routledge.
Thompson, M. E. and Watkins, B. *Dyslexic Teaching Handbook*, Whurr.
Welchman, M. *Suggestions for helping the Dyslexic Child in the Home*, Better Books.
West, T. G. *In the Mind's Eye*, Promenenthus Books.
Young, P. and Tyre, C. *Specific Learning Difficulties: A Staff Development Book*, QED, Lichfield, Staffordshire.

Literacy

Alston, J. *Spelling Helpline*, Dextral Books.
Alston, J. and Taylor, J. *Handwriting Helpline*, Dextral Books.
Goswami, U. (ed.) 'Recent Work on Reading and Spelling Development' (in *Dyslexia, Integrating Theory and Practice*, Snowling and Thomson (ed.), Whurr.
* Hulme, C. and Snowling, M. (eds) *Reading Development and Dyslexia*, Whurr.
Irlen, H. *Reading by the Colours*, Avery Publishing.
Pollock, J. *Signposts to Spelling*, Heinemann.

* Pumfrey, P. and Elliot, C. *Children's Difficulties in Reading and Writing*, Falmer Press.
Reason, R. and Boote, R. *Helping Children with Reading and Spelling: A Special Needs Manual*, Routledge.
Stirling, E. *Help for the Dyslexic Adolescent*, St David's College, Llandudno.
Thomson, M. and Watkins, E. J. *Dyslexia: A Teaching Handbook*, Whurr.

Numeracy and Other Subjects

Chinn, S. J. and Ashcroft, J. R. *Mathematics for Dyslexics: A Teaching Handbook*, Whurr.
Gilroy, D. *Applying to Higher Education for Dyslexic Students*, Dyslexia Unit, Bangor University.
Griffiths, D. and Childs, G. *Teaching Modern Languages to Pupils with Specific Learning Difficulties (Dyslexia)*, Tameside Education Centre, Lakes Road, Dukinfield, Tameside SK16 4TR.
Henderson, A. *Mathematics and Dyslexia*, St David's College, Llandudno.
Miles, T.R. and Miles, E. (eds) *Dyslexia and Mathematics*, Routledge.
Oglethorpe, S. *Instrumental Music for Dyslexics*, Whurr.
Sharma, M. *Dyscalculia and Other Learning Problems*.

Resources for Dyslexic Children

This list is not comprehensive. There is a multitude of resources aimed specifically at dyslexic children. Most programmes and materials which are aimed at non-dyslexic children are also suitable, handled sensitively and appropriately. We have restricted ourselves here to the programmes which we have found to be most useful in our teaching.

Anne Arbor Publishers Ltd (Anne Arbor, PO Box 1, Belford, Northumberland NE70 7JX — large range of dyslexic materials and books).
Augur, J. and Briggs, S. *The Hickey Multi-Sensory Teaching System*, Whurr.
Better Books (Better Books, 3 Paganel Drive, Dudley DY1 4AZ — probably the main supplier of books on the subject of dyslexia — catalogue available).
Bramley, W. *Developing Literacy for Study and Work*, Dyslexia Institute.
Brand, V. *Remedial Spelling: Spelling Made Easy*, Egon.
Cotterell, G. *The Phonic Reference File*, LDA.
Cowling, K. and Cowling, H. *Toe by Toe* (available from 8 Green Road, Basildon, West Yorks BD17 5HL).
Cripps, C. *Stile: Spelling Programme*, LDA.
Cripps, C. and Peters, M. *The Hand for Spelling Dictionary*, LDA.
Griffiths, E. *O Gam i Gam* (resource pack designed to meet to need of Welsh-speaking dyslexic children), University of Wales, Aberystwyth.
Hornsby, B. *Alpha to Omega* (4th edn), Heinemann.
Cooke, A. *Tackling Dyslexia the Bangor Way*, Whurr.
Gillingham, A. and Stillman, B. *Remedial Training for Children with Specific Learning Disabilities in Reading, Writing and Penmanship*, Cambridge Education.
LDA Living and Learning (Duke Street, Wisbech, Cambridge PE13 2AE — large range of dyslexia materials).
Miles, E. *The Bangor Dyslexia Teaching System*, Whurr.
Moseley, D. *ACE Spelling Dictionary*, LDA.

National Listening Library (for an reasonable annual fee you can borrow talking books).
Reid, G. *Specific Learning Difficulties (Dyslexia), A Handbook for Student Practice*, Moray House
TRTS (Teaching Reading Through Spelling, PO Box 1349, Wrexham LL14 4ZA) *Teaching Reading Through Spelling.*

Software for Dyslexics

There is a huge amount of software for dyslexic children. It is constantly being changed, added to and updated. In the UK nearly every county has a specialist advisory teacher with expertise in appropriate software for children with special needs. We would suggest that you contact this person for advice. You will reach him or her via the Director of Education for the county concerned. Alternatively you can contact a local British Dyslexia Association Computer Coordinator. Their addresses and contact numbers ae included in the latest *Dyslexia Handbook* (BDA, see General Reading Booklist). Below we give you a small sample of the range of mateial available. Each one is taken from the *Dyslexia Handbook for 1998*.

CALSC (Communication and Learning Skills Centre, 131, Homefield Park, Sutton SM1 2DY) *Mastering Memory* (claims to improve children's memory skills by explicit teaching of memory strategies).

Clifford, V. and Miles, M. (IANSYST, White House, 72, Fen Road, Cambridge, CB4 1UN) *Acceleread/Accelewrite: Guide to the Talking Computer Project* (claims to develop reading and writing skills using talking word-processors and structured phonic sentences).

Dyslexia Unit, Bangor (Psychology Department, University College of Wales, Bangor, Gwynedd LL57 2DG) *Dyslexia Software* (a detailed, multi-sensory programme based on structured wordlists and adopting a multi-sensory approach).

Hornsby, B. and Shear, F. (National Course Director, PO Box 535, Bromley, Kent BR1 2YF) *Touch-type, Read and Spell* (this program is based on the established *Alpha to Omega* scheme (see Resources); it enhances reading and writing skills, through touch-typing skills).

Useful Addresses

Once again we have restricted ourselves to the few addresses which we think you will find to be the most useful. Some of these are on the Internet. Check also our list of websites which follows.

Adult Dyslexia Organisation (ADO), 336 Brixton Road, London, SW9 7AA. Tel: 0171 737 7646; Helpline: 0171 924 9559.

AFASIC: The Association for all Speech Impaired Children, 374 Central Markets, Smithfield, London, EC1A 9NH. Tel: 0181 661 0877.

Arts Dyslexia Trust, c/o Lodge Cottage, Braborne Lees, Ashford, Kent, TN 25 6QZ. Tel: 01303 813221.

Bangor Dyslexia Unit, Department of Psychology, University of Bangor, Gwynedd, North Wales LL57 2DG. Tel: 01248 351151.

British Dyslexia Association, 98 London Road, Reading RG1 5AU. Tel: 01734 662677; Fax: 01734 351927; Helpline: 0118 966 8271.

Communication and Learning Skills Centre, 131, Homefield Park, Sutton, Surrey SM1 2DY. Tel: 0181 642 4663.

Dyslexia Institute, 133 Gresham Road, Staines, Middlesex TW18 2AJ. Tel: 01784 463851.

Dyslexia Association of Ireland, Suffolk Chambers, Suffolk Street, Dublin. Tel: 1 670026.
European Dyslexia Association, 3530 Royse, Norway.
Helen Arkell Dyslexia Centre, Frensham, Farnham, Surrey GU10 3BW. Tel: 01252 792400.
Hong Kong Dyslexia Association, Third Floor, 8 Crown Terrace, Pokfulam, Hong Kong. Tel: 01784 463851.
Hornsby International Dyslexia Centre, Glenshee Lodge, 262, Trinity Road, London SW18 3SN. Tel: 0181 874 1844.
Moray House Institute, Heriot Watt University, Holyrood Road, Edinburgh, EH8 AQ. Tel: 0131 558 6381.
Scottish Dyslexia Association, Unit 3, Stirling Business Centre, Wellgreen Place, Stirling, FK8 2DZ. Tel: 01786 451720.

Websites

There is a wealth of information on dyslexia on the Internet. At the time of writing when asked to search for websites containing the word 'dyslexia' the Internet came up with 4,721 entries. Our list of useful Websites begins with an extended description of the one we found most helpful, which is maintained by the British Dyslexia Association. The best approach, however, is simply to browse until you find what you need. There is a complete diversity of websites, from those which are highly erudite and academic to others which are simply dyslexic people taking the opportunity to talk to others. The following is just to give you a brief flavour of the range and diversity available.

The British Dyslexia Association (http://www.bda-dyslexia.org.uk/)
  Helpline: e-mail: info@dyslexiahelp-bda.demon.co.uk)
  This very helpful and informative site contains information on pages headed: Index to BDA Information Sheets; Publications; Local dyslexia associations; Parents, including pre-school pointers; Teachers and all in education; Adult dyslexia in college, employment and job-hunting; Computers, hardware and software for dyslexic users.
Dyslexia Institute Homepage (http//www.dyslexia-inst.org.uk/index.htm)
  Contains information about dyslexia services, dyslexia training, teaching and publication details and contact details.
The Dyslexia Page (http://www.echonyc.com/-mvidal/dyslexia/)
  Described as 'some interesting sources of information about dyslexia that I have found on the Internet'.
Dyslexia (http://lifematters.co/messagespar/131.html)
  This site asks parents of dyslexic children to contact its author.
Dyslexia My Life: an Autobiography by Girard Sagmiler (http://www.qni.com/-girards)
  Information for people with dyslexia and learning difficulties.
Bookstore — Dyslexia (http://www.ldanatl.org/stor/LD_Dyslexia.html)
  The homepage of a major supplier of educational equipment and materials for dyslexic children.
Dyslexia, The Gift (http://www.dyslexia.com)
  This site aims to 'explore the positive talents that give rise to dyslexia, and share knowledge about the best ways for dyslexic people to learn'.

Adult Dyslexia Association (http:/unix.hensa.ac.uk/ftp/pub/dyslexia/groups/contacts.
general.bib)
This is a support organisation run by adult dyslexics.
University of Wales Dyslexia Unit, Bangor (http://www.journals.wiley.com/wilcat-bin/
ops/ID0607716/1076-9242/prod)
The aim is to review and report authoritative studies of dyslexia related to intervention
programmes and professional developments.

More Local Information

We would suggest that you also find out the following information and record it
somewhere handy; maybe here:

Manager of the Local branch of British Dyslexia Association and/or Dyslexia Institute

Headteacher of school

Special Needs Co-ordinator for the School

Special Needs Governor for the school

Director of Education

Senior Special Needs Officer for the County

Principal Educational Psychologist

Educational Psychologist for school

Head of Learning Support Service

School Doctor

Head of Speech and Language Therapy Service

Index

Only the main references are given for words such as 'reading', 'spelling', 'writing' and 'memory' which occur throughout the text. Other words such as 'dyslexia' itself or 'schools' appear too often to list.